I0026714

Orasyon
Meditation

Orasyon
Meditation

A Warrior's Path To Enlightenment

DATU SHISHIR INOCALLA

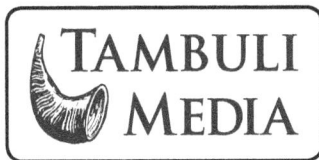

TAMBULI
MEDIA

www.TambuliMedia.com
Spring House, PA USA

DISCLAIMER

The author and publisher of this book DISCLAIM ANY RESPONSIBILITY over any injury as a result of the techniques taught in this book. Readers are advised to consult a physician about their physical condition before undergoing any strenuous training or dangerous physical activity.

First Tambuli Media Edition, October 6, 2017.
ISBN-13: 978-1-943155-29-3
ISBN-10: 1-943155-29-1

Drawings by Roger Gerhardt
Photography by Jay Cruz, Rey Merkel & Trula O'Haire
2017 Cover by Summer Bonne

DEDICATION

I would like to dedicate this book to my spiritual guru, Shrii Shrii Ananda Murthi, for showing me the path, and for his continuous guidance,

To my wife, Trula O'Haire and my son, Jesse Gautam, for their support and affection,

To the memory of my parents and the Inocalla family,

To my Arnis teacher, Professor Remy Presas, and... to all the students of Filipino Martial Arts,

To all the seekers who may see light through this book, and to Thomas H. Smith for editing, suggestions and preparation of the manuscript.

TABLE OF CONTENTS

FOREWORD

Meditative practices were developed thousands of years ago, in countries like Tibet, China, and India. The various practices made their way West and eventually grabbed the interest of mind-body enthusiasts and psychologists. Today, meditation is gaining ground as perhaps the best overall non-medical practice for self-development and promotion of well-being.

Recent research from Harvard shows that practicing meditation regularly for as little as eight weeks can cause beneficial physiological structural changes in the brain's grey matter. This is important because most of the brain's neural cell bodies are found within grey matter, which itself encompasses regions of the brain that effect sensory perception (sight and sound), muscle control, memory, emotions, auditory functions and how we make decisions and apply self-control. In other words, this is amazing proof of the power of meditation to positively affect almost every aspect of your wellbeing.

Stress is a slow and silent killer. Pent up anger and frustration and anxiety wreak havoc on the body and mind, stealing joy and happiness from daily life and shortening life span. When we hold onto stress and tension it can lead to feelings of depression, but today's exercise — an easy breathing exercise and stretch combination — will help alleviate that. It only takes a few minutes and can be done in your office, at home or at the park. Just a few moments of self-care can relieve stress and make your days much better.

Yoga and meditation practices have been shown to reduce stress and anxiety, to quiet the mind and slow the breath, and to prolong quality of life. All of this, and more, is presented in this little gem of a book by my good friend, Datu Shishir Inocalla.

In *Orasyon Meditation*, which I am proud to bring back into print as a Tambuli Media edition, Datu Shishir merges his vast experience in Indian Yoga and Filipino Orasyon meditation into a program for developing as a peaceful warrior in mind, body and spirit.

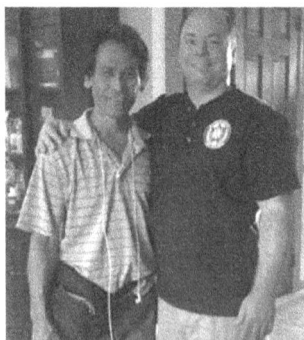

Dr. Mark Wiley
Publisher, Tambuli Media
Contributor,
Easy Health Options

I.

INTRODUCTION

Self-discipline, internal strength, peace of mind, fulfill-ment, self realization or victory... this is the Warrior's Path to Enlightenment. A warrior's way is a shortcut to his/her destiny. By concentrating on one's energy and continuously striving for victory, we make a path toward harmony, in spite of conflict. We attain peace through our struggle. For a warrior, the contest itself is the essence of life. Without struggle, there is no life.

Orasyon/meditation is a discipline for every warrior, designed to strengthen and balance his or her body, mind and spirit, and to prepare for the lifetime "battles". Internal discipline and fighting spirit will have to be desired, and, ultimately achieved. Martial Arts discipline has been the warrior's path since time immemorial. The offensive and defensive movement, the foot work and the hand motions are symbols of the warrior's ancient art. Of much greater importance are the mental strategies, the concentration and the orasyon/meditation.

It is the spiritual dimension that ultimately creates a true warrior. "Never stop until the goal is reached. Continue to fight until there is life. Move forward and never retreat. Use your body... use your mind... use your spirit. Conquer the enemy within yourself. There is only one goal... that is to find *harmony* and *peace.*"

There are many forms of meditation to consider, including Zen, Bulong, Orasyones, Dasal, Yoga, Tibetan and Christian, Taoist and relaxation meditation, to name just a few. We will certainly become confused, if we attempt to follow all the different forms of meditation or even begin to read about meditation as a complete subject. It is only through practicing a single form that we will come to understand and appreciate the benefits of meditation.

The process itself is simple. It is a matter of disciplining ourselves to meditate, practicing regularly, two times each day, for a period of 20 to 30 minutes. However, at the beginning, we may find this difficult. This book has been written to assist all meditation practitioners in the path of Martial Arts, the warrior path. Hopefully, this writing will clarify the mystery of meditation/orasyon, and will make things easier for both the beginner and the advanced practitioner.

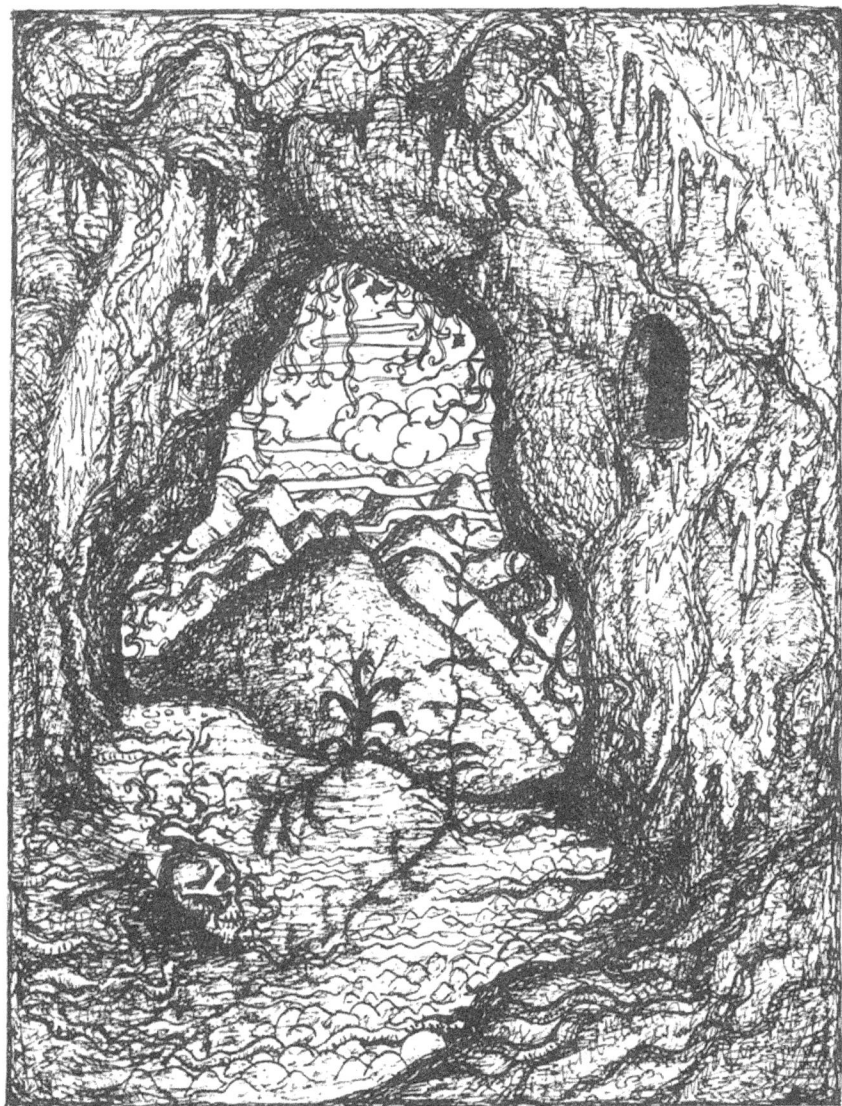

Roger Gerhardt ©

Search

II.

IN SEARCH OF THE MASTER

I was twelve and a half when I finally decided I had enough of my street life in the Philippines. I realized that I had to change my lifestyle and search for the truth, in order to lead a righteous life. I learned about a master who would teach me Orasyon/Dasal meditation and simplicity of life and I decided to follow in his footsteps.

I abandoned all my street friends and my family, and became a boy-helper for an Indian yogi. His lifestyle amazed me. He wore only orange garments, owning never more than two sets of clothes at any time. He engaged himself in teaching meditation and yogic practices to people, throughout day and night. He lived only through donations from his students. This man was a pure vegetarian and maintained chastity. The yogi was truly dedicated to his teaching. I was so impressed, I decided to follow him wherever he travelled, to learn from him, becoming a permanent student.

I am still terrified by my memories of my street life. I hold no good thoughts for my Martial Arts instructor to whom I had dedicated my years of Martial Arts training, only to be a better street fighter! Basically, and unfortunately, to survive in the street is the sole purpose of most Martial Arts training, even today.

After a few weeks under the guidance of the yogi, I began to realize that fighting was not the only goal of a true Martial Artist. It became clear to me that *meditation* was also a form of discipline. Even though it is non-violent, it is valuable to the Spirit of a Warrior. I remember my first meditation, and, how at that moment, I felt peace within me. I began to understand why my parents had taught me orasyones and prayers, to be done each evening, when I was a small boy. I suddenly missed the security of my parents and the love of God that they taught me.

It was only when I moved to Manila with my brothers and sisters, that I knew I had to become tough to survive. Of course, I now realize that being strong or "tough" doesn't mean fighting opponents, either physically or mentally. It does mean being prepared at all levels, especially in the spirit, to become a truly strong warrior. It is accepting of the law of nature and doing the best that one can in all situations that is important.

This is the strength that I have found in the master, a man of peace, but a warrior in all aspects. He spoke about righteousness and standing up for one's principles. My respect for this man is even higher today, for I see more clearly that he was a fighter for justice and the needy. He reminds me of the legendary Filipino warriors in the distant past. These ancient men were known to have prayers such as Orasyones, Agimats, Birtud (Amulet) and (Tagalimas). They were said to have been Filipino masters who had fought for their freedom. It was known that these people could only be found through an "Ermitanyo", (hermit) who had an extraordinary knowledge. I am sure that my Yogi was a living Ermitanyo. I found a Master that was a living example of his teaching. The months of living with the teacher taught me a great deal of self-discipline and inner peace.

I have had some powerful experiences that I cannot easily interpret. There was one occasion, during midnight orasyon, when I felt a total bliss and knew that I had reached a certain stage of higher consciousness. I was aware of my surroundings, but felt my entire concentration of mind was focused on a light in my forehead. My body felt light and quite numb, but I experienced no discomfort. In fact, my orasyon was so real, I could almost visualize the subject that I was concentrating on. I sat still for long hours, until very early in the morning. At this stage, I felt that it was time to return to my normal consciousness. When I woke up, one of my friends told me that I had been in my orasyon position for four hours. They were worried, because I had not moved for so long a time. Apparently, I was well-covered with large mosquitoes, yet I felt none of them bite me. All I can remember is that I had been repeating my orasyones (incanted words for meditation.) A light seemed to glow in my forehead. Afterwards, I felt so released, I felt like meditating even longer. That experience was something very extraordinary.

I discontinued my Martial Arts training and led a life of non-violence. I was content to do only my spiritual training in meditation and to serve my new master.

I was associating frequently with the master's well-to-do students, and one day I heard them talking about their incredible visit with a guru in India. I was confused, because I was happy with my present master (guru) and could not understand why another guru would be mentioned. This Indian teacher was the guru of my own master! The students told me that anyone could become like my teacher, provided that they travel to India and train directly under the Grand Master. The students felt that I could be their Filipino representative, for I had the necessary qualifications, the Acharya training, (teacher-by-example).

I was not sure whether or not I was ready for this step. I went to see my own master and told him what I had heard. My teacher was pleased to hear what I told him. He showed me a picture of an ordinary-looking man whom he called BABA. He spoke very highly of this guru and told me that it was true that he, himself, was merely a disciple of this great master living in India. He also told me he thought I was very young to meet the Grand Master. However, he said that, if my parents would give me permission, it would be alright to travel. He said that I had already learned all he could teach me and that it was time for me to learn from the highest authority. The master told me that I could also become like himself, a master. Being only thirteen years old, I was both confused and flattered by these words.

I returned to my parents in the countryside and announced that I was leaving for India. I would abandon my country and my family to become a truly universal man. My parents not only exploded with anger, they were reminded once more that my brothers and sisters had also followed my footsteps, leading a meditative lifestyle. Although we underwent a very heated discussion, my mind was already made up. I had to go to India and become an Acharya (teacher).

There were three of us from the Philippines who would become the first from my country to train in this rigorous yogic life. I had never flown anywhere before and I was both excited and very frightened by the anticipation. All my friends wished me the best and my guru gave me his blessings for my trip.

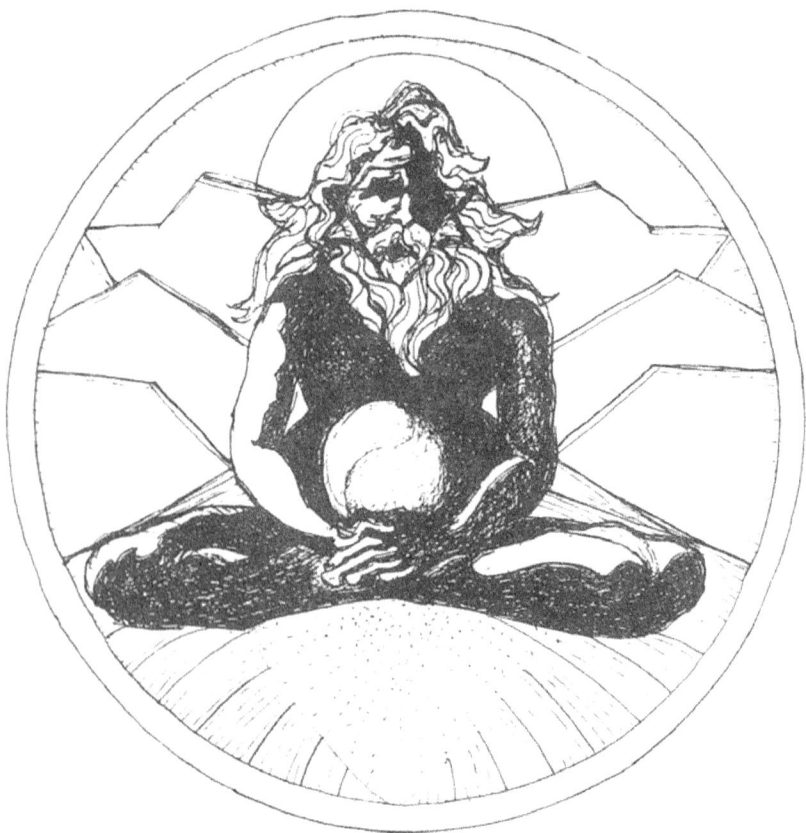

THE GRAND MASTER

The flight was long and tiring, and, as I stepped off the plane, I was totally overwhelmed by the change in the environment. I had never seen such poverty in my life. The streets of Calcutta were worse, by far, than our slums and market places in the Philippines. People – human beings – were and are actually living in rough shelters on the street comers, these unfortunates without food or the barest necessities of life. However, my attention was very much focused on finding the Master BABA.

When I reached the Master's center, I saw not merely a dozen orange-robed monks and nuns, but fifty or more. I now realized that my teacher in the Philippines was only one of hundreds of Master Babas' disciples. I was all the more intrigued to meet him. The Great Master's disciples gathered around every evening, chanting and dancing in circles, singing "Baba nam kevalam". Only the name of the Supreme Father was more hallowed.

Being so young, I was suspicious of him. I had a difficult time understanding how he had such power over so many disciples. He looked to me like an average "family" man. Although he sat in his white robe and gazed toward the sky, he was listening and watching everyone as they moved and chanted about him. When I looked at him, he seemed to be staring at me. He was smiling as if he were welcoming me home. I remember, finally, joining in with the disciples and our chant and dance became so intense that a few of my colleagues drifted into "samadhi", a spiritual trance. Their bodies became light, they cried in bliss and actually floated in the air like feathers blown by the wind. I was shock ed by the power generated by this spiritual congregation.

On one occasion, when I at last had a chance to see the Master in person, (a rare visit), I entered his room to find him sitting on his bench. Because I was nervous, I started talking rapidly, without much thought. I was afraid to tell him what was in my mind. The Master smiled and asked me a question that was deeply personal. I did not want to tell him the answer. He asked me again and I broke into tears. Suddenly, I had a clear vision of myself doing exactly what I *was* doing – crying profusely. I felt an incredible energy coming from the Master, my body became numb and I felt my hair standing up. My head "expanded" and I found myself shouting his name through my tears.

I was not aware of my surroundings. I felt my entire body floating in space. I could see no beginning nor end. I was not sure ho w long I was in that state, however, after a while, Guru Baba told me to return to "myself" and settle down. He explained to me that I had been in a spiritual trance, that he had accepted me to become his student and that he would become my master. He took away my negative karma (action and reaction). He told me that my energy was now going to be focused in purifying myself, helping the needy and becoming a spiritual warrior. He said that I had an important mission ahead of me and he assured me that, wherever I was, he would also be there. Nor should I be afraid. I would be trained and guided by him personally, where ever I was now and would ever go in this world.

I was still mesmerized when I left his room. I felt very fortunate and full of energy (that would last over a long period), and yet I did not really understand what had happened, how or why. All I knew was that I had found a true Grand Master.

After my first contact with the teacher, I continued to feel at peace and to recognize the energy that he had passed on to me. However, even after a few weeks, I was still unsure of what was happening to me, and also, whether or not I should dedicate my whole being to this new mission.

Acharya training means undertaking long and rigorous yogic discipline in the monastery. It was easier for me to give up a great deal than it was for the older boys, because I was only fourteen, with no real commitments. However, after living so freely in the streets of Manila, I was not sure whether or not I was ready to dedicate my life to such an arduous training.

Not many weeks later, I attended one of the largest spiritual gatherings ever held in Calcutta. There were thousands of disciples waiting to hear the Master's words. Everyone was singing and dancing, and the Guru Baba gave an hour-long talk. When he had finished, everyone was silent. He look ed up at the sky and gave a powerful mudra (spiritual gesture). Guru Baba delivered a tremendous Khi-lakas (energy) to thousands of his students. I was in the middle of the crowd and I watched the microphone he was using sway back and forth, as if there was a strong wind wielding it from side to side. Row by row, the students fell backward, as if they were struck by a bolt of strong energy.

They all fell into a spiritual trance, calling his name. I had never before witnessed this tremendous energy. My studies in Martial Arts never mentioned that such incredible energy could be manifested by a single individual. I had only read about super-human feats and never expected to witness such power. Guru Baba was a living example of this amazing energy.

I looked back upon my Martial Arts and realized that I was now pursuing the very same goals; speed, power and the lifetime of training necessary for mastery of the arts. All this training could lead to inner strength, peace of mind and self-realization. (T he fighting techniques, Balisong, sticks and other forms, are all geared to self-discipline and contentment.) Here were these monks who were non-violent, who didn't practice martial arts, who meditated and purified themselves... achieving the same goals!

They succeeded in purifying themselves more quickly than the y could have using the martial arts way, because they did not develop the inflated ego that is demanded by many of the "martial arts" schools. Their simple orasyon technique led to the same goal. With this realization, I decided that I would have to enter the monastery and become a monk.

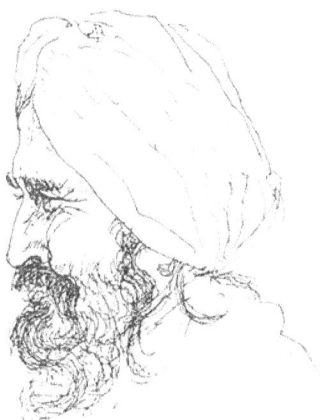

Monk

THE MONASTERY

A small, four-bedroom stone house was our training center for monks. It was so crowded, we had to sleep side by side like rows of sardines. There was only one toilet for all the trainees and there were fifty of us in the small house. We arose at four o'clock in the morning and meditated for two hours, the first of four sessions during the day. We did exercises and yogic postures. During the first three weeks, I was in a room with an electric fan, which helped to cool me in the 110° F heat. After a while, I was transferred into a bigger room without a fan, and would remain there until I graduated. My concern grew when I heard about someone who had resided there for years and still had not passed upward to the level of teacher.

There were also a few who stayed for only a few months, managing to pass in that short time, but more often, students could not stand the rigorous training and dropped out altogether. Nonetheless, I was very determined to succeed. I felt that all the hardship was but a test of my dedication and sincerity. From morning until bedtime, we studied Eastern Philosophy, different languages and social philosophy. These were interspersed with hours of meditation and memorization of Sanskrit prayers.

My two Filipino friends took sick after a few months in residence and left for home. I was sad, because they were the only ones with whom I could speak Filipino. They also "covered" for me when I sneaked out and jumped over the high wall to run to the market for soft drinks and chocolate!

I had been studying very hard and was becoming desperate, wishing now to graduate at the earliest possible moment. Every week, new people and old trainees came and went like the tide. I had memorized all my lessons, however, at exam time, held every three months, the trainers would call me to the examining room, but never asked me to answer any of their questions. I remember leaving the room very angrily, knowing that I failed the exam again without a chance to prove myself. They must have known that I was not ready. I usually returned to my quarters and punched the concrete wall out of frustration. This reaction was not exactly the one I was being taught by my trainers!

There was one particular type of training in which we became beggars, to teach us humility. We had only a single white cloth to wrap around us and we carried a wooden begging bowl. We were not allowed to speak, except to say "Hare-om-tat sat", (God is the Universe). We begged for our food and we did not eat, if we were unsuccessful.

I recall being chased by dogs and being humiliated by passers-by, especially the store owners. At the same time, there were people who were very kind. At times I had to protect myself against the dogs, using an Arnis walking stick. However, I grew more confident each day.

Occasionally, around three in the morning, I slipped out to the park and practiced my Martial Arts. Although I realized that I was supposed to feel at home in the monastery, Martial Arts training was something I missed and I wanted to relive those experiences. After a while, some of my fellow students also joined me in my private training sessions.

I remember once growing sick and feeling totally weak. I grew so helpless, I wanted to let go of all my fears and anxieties. One night, while everyone else was sleeping, I began to meditate as I watched the picture of my master, Baba. It was at this moment that I totally surrendered my energies and thoughts to the master. At once, I felt peaceful, and, for the first time, felt at home. Time and reputation were no longer important to me. Simply enjoying what I was doing became my only concern and I then began, and continued, to purify myself.

Finally, I was called to sit for the examination once again. This time, I let go of my expectations. I knew that I would pass when I was ready. In the examination room, I was asked only one very simple question. I was very surprised, because I had expected a more difficult quizzing. After a few hours, the examiner announced that I had passed the training. I could not believe that I had at last completed my early training, after one and a half years of work and meditation in that small monastery. I knew now that when we were ready, we would be called. When we were ready, the master would come. It was true that the master was within us all. Learning is a reflection of the master.

FAREWELL TO THE MASTER

I was so happy to know that, in spite of my age, (15 years), I actually completed the monastic training. I was called to go to Patna, India, for field experience. I would have to put my long training into practice. At this time, I was appointed to be an assistant in charge of twelve children in an orphanage. My work was more active than prayerful, having to beg and ask for donations for the children in my care. Often riding my bicycle for miles, I went door to door, asking for food supplies for my children. It was very hard sometimes, especially during the winter months, wrapped in a single blanket, riding a bicycle very early in the morning in freezing temperatures and driving rain. I would go from village to village, sometimes being turned away, although most people were sympathetic. A few would stone me, because they thought that, my being a monk, I was holding the children captive in order that they too would become monks!

Sometimes the food was stale when we received it. Often, the bread had to be toasted immediately, so that it would not rot any further. I had never seen such poverty and starvation in my life, but I felt now that I was one with the sufferers.

We also ran a day-care school for these young boys. I had to learn quickly, because two of the students were almost my age and they might have felt that they should not obey me. It was hard enough for me to adjust to their culture, let alone to handle an orphanage for young people. But, miraculously, beyond all this poverty and hardship, I felt I was actually doing some good for my charges. I felt that my spiritual life was progressing.

Compared to my life on the streets of Manila, this existence was less severe. I was no longer constantly threatened. I had surrendered myself to my mission and to my master. I didn't worry about my future or the dangers that might await me. In reality, my life as a monk was probably harder than my previous times, but the difference was, I now felt joy and contentment. Every afternoon, I could visit my master. I attended all his discourses and meditation/orasyon. He often joked with me, saying, "Where is the little boy, Shishir?" Sometimes he asked me to sit near him or requested me to dance the Tandava (warrior dance). I was very fortunate to be so accepted by the master. I had nothing more to ask for. I was fulfilled.

I had never dreamed of leaving the master for any reason. The life of a disciple *is* his master. This can be demonstrated by recalling one special time, when we celebrated the arrival of the New Year. We usually had a big gathering at which the master gave us new programs and gave his blessing to everyone.

While organizing this big event, I heard terrible news. My superior wanted me to leave immediately, together with some of my brother monks, to go to Bangladesh to start relief work for the war victims. I had never thought of leaving the master. I was very sad and thought of appealing to my superiors to allow me to remain at my group home. While I was busy thinking of all the possible excuses to stay, I heard some of my monk brothers talking in anguish, while others were angry and warlike. I quickly learned that the reason for our journey was that our beloved master had been arrested by the Indian authorities for totally false charges, all political in nature. His "crime" consisted of his criticism of the government for its corruption!

Baba was not allowed to have any visitors and was confined in jail. There was incredible anger in the air. We were all ready to die for the master, but the instructions from my superior were to continue our given work. I was assigned to leave the next day.

That night I did not sleep. I would follow my posting, but I wanted to see the master before I left. I wanted to have his blessings. I remembered the great saying of the lord, Christ, "Knock, and the door shall be opened unto you. Ask, and it shall be given unto you." I decided to meditate all night, until I had a vision of my master. I needed his blessing before I went anywhere. I knew that, when a devotee asked his master, the master could not refuse. This is one weakness of the master.

I began to meditate around nine in the evening. Many hours passed by and I was falling asleep. My back and feet were aching but I had no doubt that the master would appear. I kept reminding myself of the lord Buddha, sitting under a banyan tree for days and nights, until, finally, he attained his enlightenment. I called my master. I called his presence. At four in the morning, I heard my monk brothers shouting and jumping with joy. "Master Baba is here!"

I was totally shocked. I woke up from my calm state and leaped around with happiness. I immediately joined my brother monks. They said that the master was ill, and that the authorities were taking him to a nearby hospital for medical help. I knew that my master had heard my call. Surely enough, in a matter of a few hours, the master was sitting on the veranda of the hospital, smiling to all his disciples. I was quite content to watch him from a distance, until one disciple grabbed me and urged me to follow him, because guru Baba was being transferred to another medical building. He would be walking outside the building and we would have a chance to say "Pranam", a gesture of paying respect. I would at last receive my blessing.

Baba actually came down to the lawn and simultaneously we bowed and received the blessing from him. Amazingly, the police escort around him was sympathetic. They were also enjoying his blessing. I told my master that I was posted to Bangladesh to do relief work for the victims of war. Baba gave me a broad smile and told me to continue my good works. He also said that, where ever I was, he would also be there. At those simple words, a half-dozen of us fell at his feet. We cried out and called his name.

I left shortly for Bangladesh to begin a new set of experiences, once more opening my eyes to the world that lay await for me. And my Master, Guru Baba? His world swiftly closed upon him, just as mine was expanding. But that was the way.

Another time, another volume to be written. The pathway of our lives, my humble existence, and the brilliant way of the master Baba, will both unfold at the next patient telling.

THE ROLE OF THE MASTER

In Tantric tradition, a guru is necessary to guide the students or disciples. Tantrika is one of the most difficult paths to enlightenment. This was developed by lord Shiva, around 6500 B.C., in India. It is a warrior's way of liberation through struggle. The student attains realization or enlightenment through clash or struggle. It is most definitely a quick way to fulfillment, but, due to its intensity, a guru is necessary for guidance, to make sure that the student does not go astray. In this order, an enlightened guru is the only teacher that is capable of guiding the student.

In the Philippine tradition, the passing on of the master's knowledge is almost always confined to family clans, often from father to son. A master who has "Galing", or "Birdud", (amulets), is usually a very powerful person. He is embedded in his religion, Islam or Christianity. He has "Anting-Anting" a talisman that protects him from danger, making himself invincible. He wears this amulet constantly. He places it around his neck, holds it in his mouth or ties it around his waist. He also repeats powerful orasyones and prayers. Anting-Anting or "Galing" is also applied in healing of all kinds. However, there are certain individuals who use this power for evil purposes.

There are many supernatural abilities that Filipino folks are said to have long experienced, through to the present day. These are similar to phenomena known in other countries. The Ninja in Japan, the Yogi in India, the sorcerer in Europe and the Shaman of the native Indian are all said to carry these abilities. These practices lead to the spiritual disciplines, mental powers all humans may possess. In Tantric philosophy, amazing abilities and miracles can be explained. The old masters of the East warn us that we must not be blinded by these supernatural abilities. They can be both destructive and misleading.

Self-realization, contentment and peace are the true goals in life. It is true that men who have all power and glory may not be content nor happy. It is better to be simple and unknown. If you can lead a life without requiring great recognition, it is possible to experience true contentment and peace.

III.

CONDUCT FOR
MEDITATION & ORASYON

It is necessary to follow certain principles of conduct in our daily lives. It helps us to know how to limit ourselves or develop some form of self-discipline. In this society, it is always tempting to over-extend ourselves, causing us to lose track of our direction. We either overdo, or we "slack off", we overwork or we do not work enough, we over indulge in food or we starve ourselves, we sleep too little or too much. This constant imbalance is a common cycle in our daily living. We use the excuse that "there is always tomorrow", or "it's too late". We seem to think that we must do everything now or not at all. There will always be reasons for avoiding regularity in our meditative practice as well. This is why there is a necessity for the principles of moral conduct for a meditation/orasyon practitioner.

There is an old saying, "Whatever you do to others will come back to you", and this holds true, even though it may reveal itself at some other time, in some other place.

This is the Law of KARMA. (Action and Reaction) "Whatever you plant, so shall you reap."

1. Ahim'sa – Non-Hurting – by thoughts, Words or Actions.

   Naturally, we cannot avoid becoming angry or thinking negatively of someone we know who might be taking advantage of us or hurting us in some way. However, losing our temper, our balance, is another matter. It becomes a burden to us, if we are so bothered that we cannot meditate or sleep because we are angry. We soon begin to talk and act out our anger. It is best, when we become angry, to avoid being carried away by our hurt. Being angry for good reason is a natural behavior, but be coming mean-minded is not.

   It is good to perform Dasal or meditate with a clear mind, our peace undisturbed by negative thoughts. The Martial Arts discipline is based upon the art of fighting. However, the goal is, ultimately, The Way Of Peace. It is true that a relaxed, skilled fighter will subdue a nervous, loud Samurai. As the deepness of Water is shown in its Serenity, so the depth of mind is shown in Wisdom and Clarity. There is a saying; "The Best of Warriors is the one who wins battles without waging war".

2. Satya – Truthfulness

   People who are truthful carry weight in their words and actions. Telling lies, or saying what people want to hear, instead of the reality of fact, is hiding our true nature. Later on, this weakness will affect us by building a duality of truth and untruth. We should always be truthful in our thoughts, words and actions. This will help our orasyon/meditation by allowing us to focus with deeper concentration. It will make us clearer in our perceptions.

3. Brahmacarya – Positive Awareness – seeing our thoughts words, actions and surroundings with care and a positive outlook. We must guard against protecting negativeness in ourselves and in anything about us. How we think, so we become. Appreciate and care for both the little and the greater things within ourselves and our society. There will always seem to be good and bad with in us and our surroundings, and this may take time to change, but our attitude should always be positive. We should be aware of and appreciate the fact that we are part of this creation. A healthy and positive attitude always uplifts our spirit and helps us to meditate peacefully.

4. Asteya – Non-stealing

   It is not right to take something that is not ours. It causes us to become mean-minded, and others, to act resentfully towards us. With this kind of attitude, it will be difficult for us to meditate or to pray. We might be able to run away from other people, or the law, however, our own conscience will always follow us and our feelings of guilt will disturb our inner peace. We may even have money and fame, but only through desirable action can we attain prosperity *and* peace.

5. Aparigraha – Non-Accumulation – proper utilization of wealth; balancing our needs.

   By accumulating what is necessary for us to grow and achieve our goals, we need not burden ourselves with those things that are not necessary, nor need we waste time accumulating them. To become wealthy and famous may be fine, however, better than these is happiness and self-actualization in our lifetime. The pursuit of great wealth can be a burden. It is necessary for a meditator/orasyones on the warrior path to properly utilize his efforts so that he does not lose track of his true goal. We must balance our needs: wealth and security for our body and a state of mental peace; self-realization and enlightenment for our spiritual and overall well-being.

6. Shaoca – Cleanliness – maintaining a clean mind, body and surroundings.

   A meditator or orasyon practitioner cannot clutter his or her mind with unnecessary thoughts or ideas.

Only thoughts that have meaning and purpose and are related to uplifting one's own consciousness should be maintained in the mind. Whatever you put into your mind will result in its expression. For example, if you think you will become ill and you imagine being ill, you may become ill.

The body should be healthy and clean. We cannot concentrate properly, if there is imbalance in our mind and body. When we meditate and perform orasyon, we clean the refuse from our mind and it is only natural that the body should follow a similar course. A daily bath is not only refreshing, but it releases new forces within the body. Clean and tidy clothes make us feel alive and well.

Our environment becomes our expression. (Imagine saying Dasal/ prayers or meditating in a disco pub, with loud music, background noise and action surrounding us 1.) We are affected by our surroundings, so it is necessary to maintain a clean and peaceful environment. It helps us to concentrate and meditate. A tidy office and a clean home allow us to work and relax more readily.

7. Santos'a − Contentment − simplicity and self-satisfaction.

It is good to set high goals and it is important to move toward attaining our maximum potential as human beings. At the same time, it is necessary to appreciate and to feel satisfied with our efforts. Achieving success and attaining glory is not as satisfying as the effort that we spend while working toward that goal. We should enjoy ourselves while we work rather than become so ambitious that we allow ourselves to lose our direction. The old "business theory" of never being satisfied, but always working harder and longer, is only useful for achieving short term goals, such as wealth and physical comfort. Spiritual happiness and long life arise from something simpler, and they bring with them, a feeling of appreciation and fulfillment. Balancing our desires, wealth and wisdom brings fulfillment of our needs. We should appreciate what we have and continually grow in this spirit.

8. Tapah – Service – helping others without expecting a reward in return. Meditators and orasyones strengthen and clarify their minds. They are effective and clear in their words, thoughts and actions. It is then necessary to share some of their good intentions with others who also need direction on the path. Like a candle in the dark, their light will shine naturally and illuminate the way. A person who is naturally clear shares and serves without expectation. On the other hand, one should balance the process of giving, being careful not to overdo

"good deeds". Always maintain enough strength to share and grow in all aspects of life. There will always be something we can learn.

9. Svadhyaya – Open Mindedness

Broad mindedness gives us room to grow. Life itself is continually moving. Sometimes we are up, sometimes down. It is a good practice to open ourselves to all things. We must learn about and study our weaknesses and strengths, so that we can increase our resources and become clearer in our direction.

Meditation, orasyon or bulong, simplifies our thoughts when our minds become cluttered. Opening up to new ideas and exploring new methods of being creative make life revolve on a higher and clearer plane. We are prevented from becoming bogged down. We are assured of continued growth. Meditation, dasal and orasyon all help us to center our awareness, while we grow to new understanding.

10. Iishvara – Pranidhana – Clear Direction Towards Goodness Keep in mind that we are never working alone. Some source we might term the Supreme Ki lakas, (energy), gives us the necessary strength to discover our own individual Ki lakas force, guides us along with our surroundings until, finally, we realize

our ultimate goal. Maintaining a clear idea that this Universal Force gives us guidance and continuous inspiration, helps us to be centered and confident, yet not ego-centered.

An orasyones should have in mind a clear direction and maintain this force as his strength and his guide in all his activities, knowing that, eventually, they will balance and merge with this Universal Force and become one with it. Then can we accept that everything around us is part and parcel of our inner being. This is the stage of achieving Inner Force in the warriors' path of Martial Arts that we call Khi Chi Lakas. This Inner Force is achieved only through years of training, together with recognition of the unity of mind and body.

Note: These teachings are based upon my Master, Shrii Shrii Ananda Murthi's work. I have made a few changes so that the reading might be better understood by the layman.

"A Guide To Human Conduct" published by Ananda Marga Pracaraka Samgha, Philippines, 1977.

IV.

EXERCISE AND BODY CONDITIONING

One should maintain a balanced form of mental and physical health. External exercises such as jogging, swimming, Martial Arts, Arnis, tennis and other forms of strenuous and competitive sport discipline our body and condition us for day-to-day living.

Internal exercise such as meditation, Tai-chi, Bulong, Orasyon, Aikido, yoga, nature walks, etc., are directed more toward developing our inner spiritual awareness, strengthening our inner organs and counter-balancing the stresses and pressures we experience in our daily activities in society.

Body conditioning must also include proper diet. Food affects our thoughts and actions. Vegetarian, healthy, fresh foods are thought to be more easily assimilated into our bodies. They offer sufficient energy to carry on the daily activities for an orasyones and meditator to enjoy a simple healthy diet. Healthy foods are listed in further pages. We do not need to kill higher forms of life in order that we ourselves live. However, one should not force himself to give up anything. Instead, we should strengthen our self-discipline and meditation, becoming more aware. Soon, our body and consciousness will voluntarily choose the right path for us to follow.

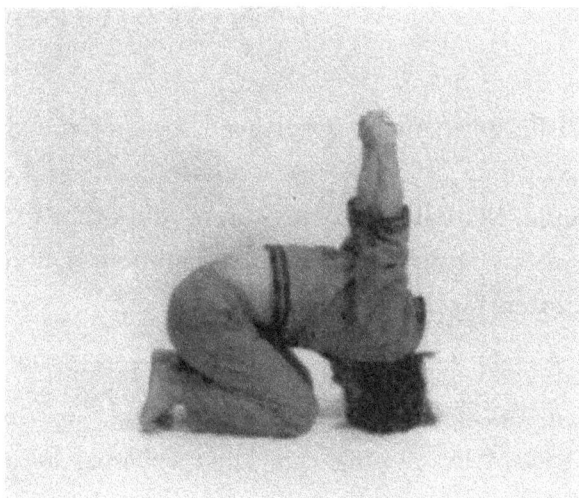

Fig 1

V

BREATHING

Fresh air and proper breathing are keys to a healthy, long life. Food, water, sunlight, etc., are necessary for life, but oxygen and proper breathing are essential for calming and centering the mind. By learning to fully circulate the air, we can achieve longevity and increase energy in the body.

We notice that a person who is very excited, angry or haggard, breathes similarly to a tired dog, rapidly and shallow, using too much energy, releasing strong emotions which tend to exhaust and shorten life.

EXERCISES FOR PROPER BREATHING

1. a) Breathe in (half – inhalation) using only the nostrils. Expand the diaphragm, then bring the rest of the air into the "stomach".

   b) Breathe in, using the nostrils, (full inhalation), bringing all the air into the chest, expanding the chest.

c) Make a full exhalation, using fingers to compress the abdominal muscles for a complete, deep breath release.

Repeat these motions six times, then, breathe normally.

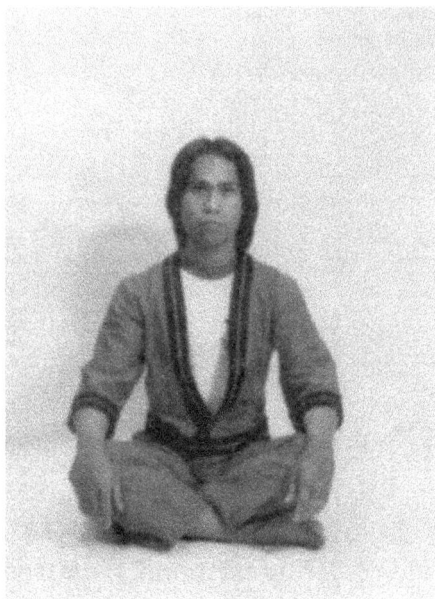

Fig 2

2. Holding Breath

    Perform the same breathing process as above, but expand and contract the abdominal and chest muscles. This second sequence involves holding the breath during every inhalation and exhalation, from 4 to 6 seconds. For example: inhale, count to 4, then exhale, holding for 4 counts. Repeat the same breathing rate, 6 to 8 times, then relax and breathe normally.

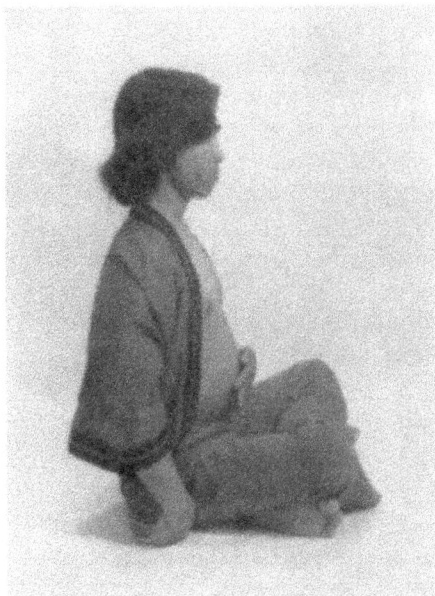

Fig 3
Inhale deeply,
supporting
diaphragm.

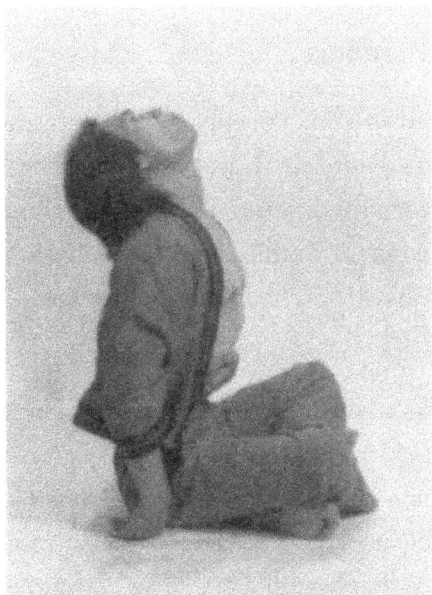

Fig 4
Tilt head back
carefully.

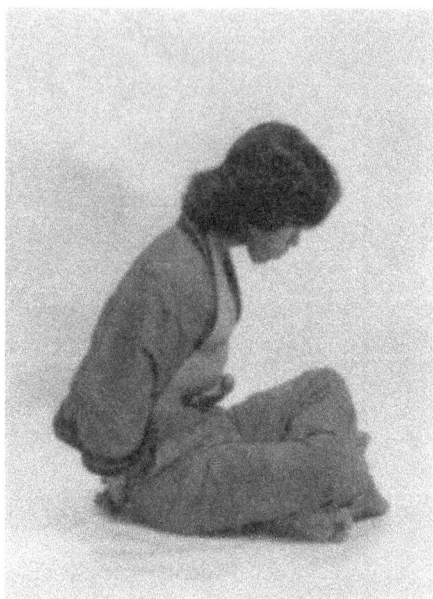

Fig 5
Tilt slowly forward,
left hand supporting
diaphragm. Exhale.

3. Ideative Singular Breathing

This is a more advanced, complicated breathing technique. First, try exercises 1 and 2 to relax and calm the mind before meditation. Practice the third technique, once you have familiarized yourself with the first two and have practiced them for one or two months.

Maintain the movement of the diaphragm and chest during each breath. Do the Holding Breath exercise, but this time, inhale only through the left nostril, blocking the right nostril with the right thumb. Hold for 4 seconds. Imagine positive energies entering your left nostril and running through every part of your body.

Exhale only through the right nostril, blocking the left nostril with the right fingertips, exhaling all the negative forces from the body. Hold for 4 seconds.

Inhale again through the right nostril by blocking the left nostril with the same fingertips and imagine the positive forces entering the right nostril and spreading throughout the body, relieving the energy blocks and tension. Hold for 4 seconds.

Exhale once more through the left nostril by blocking the right nostril with the right thumb, releasing all the negative energy in the body. Hold for 4 seconds. The sequence is:

a) Inhale left   b) Exhale right

c) Inhale right   d) Exhale left.

Perform the sequence 3 times daily (before Dasal/ meditation) for one month, and then, increase slowly, up to seven times per day, over another month. "7" times will be the maximum number of repetitions performed at any time. This is the advanced breathing technique. It would be helpful if you could practice under personal instruction by a qualified teacher.

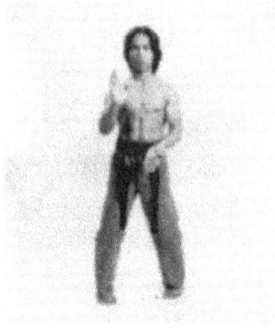

Note: Sainchin Karate breathing, using deep breathing and bodily tension, is the External Pranayam (Science of Breathing). This exercise is directed more to physical exertion and external strength. This is the true meaning of KIA to put power into your punch or kick. Breathing is the center of *Life Force*.

VI.

WITHDRAWAL

It is only after the following first three steps that we can easily practice withdrawal. Self-discipline, a healthy mind and body and proper breathing are all necessary for achieving detachment and withdrawal from our senses.

Choose a convenient place and posture for Dasal or meditation. The area must be free from distractions. Sit in a Zen, kneeling cross-legged, or in the lotus position, (finding the most relaxed posture for yourself) and maintain that position during meditation and Dasal. (See cover Illustration) Lie down, if you are very tired, or sit in a chair or on a cushion, if you feel that is necessary. You can also start by lying down and then sit up when you feel more energized. You can focus better when in a sitting position, there being less chance of falling asleep. It also limits your sense of touch.

FIRST TECHNIQUE:

1. Close your eyes or look at the tip of your nose to withdraw your vision.

2. Chant the Auma (Aumaa) sound, loud and long. "Aumaaa" continuously, until you feel withdrawn from outside your body. Chanting relaxing songs helps you to withdraw from sound.

   (Some meditation and Dasal practitioners burn incense to counter the odors in the meditation room. This helps them to withdraw from a sense of negative odors. A few meditators/orasyones rinse their mouths with water or avoid taking food 20 to 30 minutes before meditating. Advanced meditators/Bulong practitioners curl their tongues back ward to eliminate the sense of taste.)

SECOND TECHNIQUE:

1. Sitting in a cross-legged position, or kneeling, relax, closing the eyes and breathing normally. Imagine yourself alone, meditating on top of a mountain or in the middle of the sea, floating peacefully. Relaxed breathing calm. Inhale. Relax.

2. Withdraw from the outside. Imagine now a positive force around you, in the form of a white cloud moving through your legs, torso and up to your head. Feel this comfortable energy slowly entering

your entire body. Start at your toes. Imagine the light entering your right leg through your toes, shin, knee, thigh, rising up all the way up to the base of your spine. Repeat this visualization, starting with your left leg, a gentle light force from the toes, all the way to the spine. Go through this at your own speed. Relax and feel at peace.

3. From the base of the spine, feel this energy force rising up to your stomach, to your chest, all the way up to your neck. Relax every part of your internal organs, muscles and nerves. Relax and feel at peace.

4. Now feel and visualize the force entering your right arm through your fingertips, palm, wrist, forearm, elbow, upper arm, all the way to your shoulder and neck. Relax and feel at peace.

    Repeat the same process in the left arm, following the same sequence, moving at your own rate of speed. Again merge the energy forces in your neck. Relax and feel at peace.

5. Now feel the forces in your neck, rising all the way to your jaw, lips, nose and face, to your ears. Relax the back of the head, eyes, and finally, your forehead.

6. Now focus and concentrate on your forehead. Imagine a bright light of energy in your forehead. Inhale, bringing the forces into your system. Exhale,

releasing the energy, allowing it to flow outward. At this stage, there are *three* factors to remember:

1) Light in the forehead

2) Gentle Breathing

3) Relaxation

Maintain this light in your forehead, also maintaining your breathing, and then relax your entire body.

If there are any disruptive thoughts present, or if you lose your focus of attention, bring your thoughts back to the light in your forehead. Relax your breathing and feel at peace. Maintain this exercise as your process of withdrawal.

"Before you can tame a wild beast, you first have to befriend it."

Tracing your feelings through every part of your body, relaxing and focusing on the light, slows down your thoughts and gently directs them to one point. The light in your forehead is the center of your concentration.

VII.

CONCENTRATION
– FOCUSING

It is only through the withdrawal process that we can properly concentrate and focus our minds on one-pointedness. Only after subduing our five senses and successfully holding our mind in one concentrated light energy without interruption, can we actually say that we are in the stage of concentration.

It is true that we cannot shut out the world outside us. It is not our desire to control or to shut out the world. We allow it to flow as it is. However, we do not allow the world outside or inside to distract us away from our point of concentration.

It is only through a slow, gentle withdrawal process that we can attain a relaxed and natural state of concentration. Forcing ourselves to concentrate only invites headaches, pressure and impatience. Letting go of all unnecessary thoughts, visions, images, etc., and maintaining one thought, one subject a single vision, is our key to concentration.

Concentration helps us to increase our energy, clarify our direction, develop an inner strength, achieve our goals and attain both serenity and inner peace.

At this stage of concentration, only two things exist:

(1) Unit "I"

(2) Supreme "I" or light

Focus your mind, body and soul one hundred percent.

"Not a blink of an eye not a whisper in the wind."

At this point, the mental energy is very strong. It is necessary to concentrate on an idea that has an *elevated* meaning in order to direct the mental strength toward intuitive growth or spiritual awareness. Strength without direction, or wrong direction, is dangerous. This is the reason why advanced meditators are advised to use a mantra or Dasal orasyon.

Da/sal – words used for salvation.

Man/tra – "that which liberates the mind ".

FOUR CHARACTERS OF MANTRAS

1) Ideative – it has an elevating idea; uplifting, spiritual in nature,

2) Rhythmic – it connects our breathing. It flows with our inner force,

3) Incantative – it has a natural quality that attracts our mind,

4) Source – it has a living source of power.

Mantras have been developed since time immemorial and are often used by meditators as a key for unlocking their innermost potential and their understanding and knowledge. For example:

BABANAM – Supreme Consciousness only,

KEVALAM – the one and only.

This mantra was created by my master in India, Shrii Ananda Murthi. Let us use this mantra to focus our concentration Or.

DI YOS – Supreme GOD – used by Filipinos since time immemorial.

Inhale – BABANAM or DI... Exhale – KEVALAM or YOS

Repeat this process until no other thought exists in your mind.

Maintain only in your mind, BABANAM... KEVALAM.

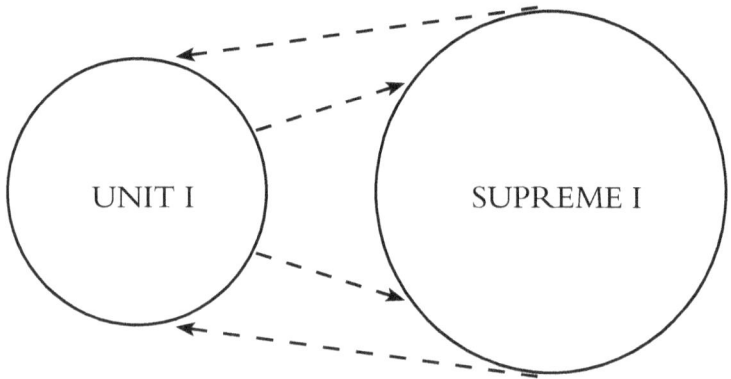

Fig 3 Concentration

VIII.

MEDITATION/ORASYON
– STATE OF EMPTY MIND

In this state, there are no thoughts, no shapes, no forms. It is the state of oneness. It is the stage where in unit mind and the Supreme Mind become one. No more separation of the ego. This is the stage when Dasal, mantra and unit mind merge into one entity. It is this state alone we call meditation or orasyon. No further separation. No further duality.

It takes preparation, practice and consistency to attain this state of consciousness. Not every time that we sit and perform Dasal, or meditate, do we attain this state. We should be satisfied just to be able to withdraw from our senses and achieve some form of concentration of mind.

Orasyon, meditation cannot be pushed. It is a very natural process of merging. It happens when we are ready. When the time is right, we experience this state of mind.

This process is similar to that experienced by a person who has spent a long time trying to find a solution to a problem. Day after day, he is engrossed in the complexity of the problem, and the more he thinks about it, the more complicated it seems to grow. Finally, after becoming completely frustrated in his attempt to press for a solution, he goes for a walk in a vast field. He feels completely at ease, the pressure leaves his mind and he becomes "unconscious" of his problem. It is at this time that the solution finally arises, and, with an "ah-hahu, he has it! It is at this stage, (the Ah-hah) where there is no word, no intention, no question or solution, that we experience intuitive meditation orasyon.

It is for this reason that a meditator/orasyones should rely upon his intuition. In this state, there are no mistakes. It is the flow of Universal Force.

Our rational mind cannot logically explain this process. We can only tidy up the clutter of our mind, maintain a regular Dasal and meditation practice, listening and slowly becoming aware of that voice within. We should trust our intuitive mind. We need to cleanse and purify our mind to nurture awareness of our actions and right consciousness. Meditate, not to find answers, practice orasyon not to be supernatural, but to empty the mind. Trusting our intuitive or meditative mind makes things simpler, because it is beyond disruption. Universal flow cannot be opposed.

Today's complexities detach us from the inner flow of the universe. Many people are out of touch with their intuitive mind and this results in great problems in their lives. Many wait until something disastrous happens before taking action. For example, when people are confined to hospital because of a major illness, only then do they realize that they should have taken care of their health.

Dasal meditation is the key to understanding our intuitive mind.

There are two stages of meditation, Dasal and orasyon:

1) Relaxation; making us feel peaceful and unstrained. It releases mental pressures, increases our energy and makes us creative.

2) Enlightenment; we realize fulfillment, simplicity, self-realization and oneness with the Universal Force.

IN DIAGRAM FORM:

STAGE ONE   STAGE TWO

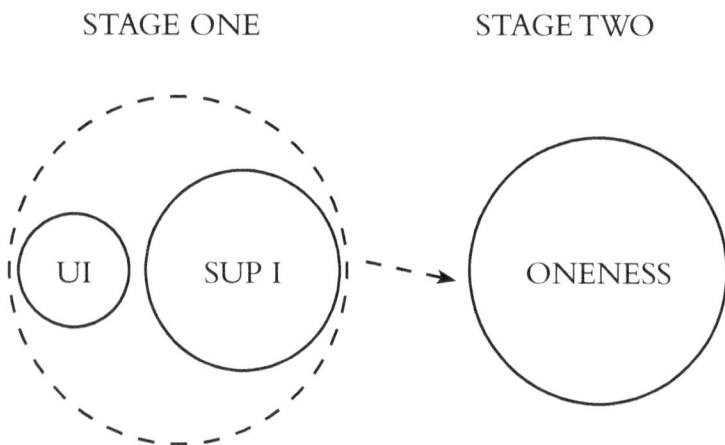

Fig 4 Meditation Merger

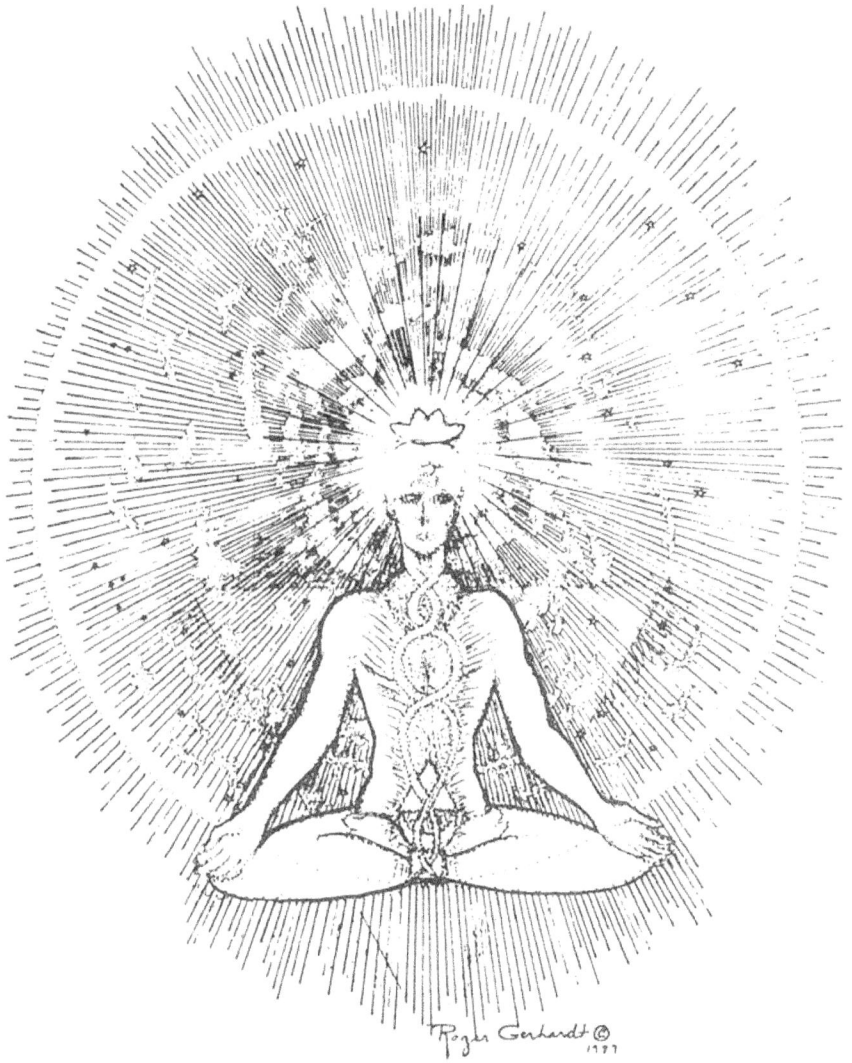

Enlightenment

IX

CLARITY
SELF-REALIZATION,
SELF-ACTUALIZATION
AND ENLIGHTENMENT.

Only after the merging of unit mind with Supreme Mind is there oneness or Empty Mind. Only through Empty Mind are clarity and realization possible.

This is the last stage of meditation, the goal of all orasyones. This is the Stage of Enlightenment or Gr ea t Understanding. Individuals who attain this state become teachers by example. Their actions speak for themselves. Individuals who attain this state become living proof of their teachings or discipline. They become True Warriors in the real essence. It is a mastery of oneself. The practitioner becomes a practical person.

Thoughts, words and actions are synchronized. There is now clarity and reality in each action performed. This is a result of Empty Mind or intuitive mind; clarity of expression through mind and body. This is the last stage of meditation orasyon. At this point we can appreciate our efforts in regular meditation and Dasal. Everything becomes clearer, and, naturally, every thing becomes more simple. In this stage, we no longer lose direction, but flow as in the highs and lows of a wave.

Of course, we are still a part of this society. It is natural to live and work and enjoy our experiences while we are able. The difference is, now we are *aware* of our actions and limits. We no longer become confused and lost. We continue to move and grow, not allowing desires and wan ts to disrupt our lives. We may have many desires, how ever, there are only a few things that we really need, and now we have a clearer understanding of what they are. Our choices can be guided by wisdom.

Clarity and Enlightenment are the goals of each and every one of us. Whether our path is religious, financial, academic, or health-oriented, we are all direct ed toward the same goal. Only the process and intensity are different. We all wish for some degree of happiness and self satisfaction, but only Clarity and Enlightenment will truly fulfill our infinite desires and satisfy our unending search.

There are stages of clarity, the degrees dependent upon what the individual wishes to attain and what preparation is required to attain it. For instance, if a businessman wants to attain wealth and prosperity, he works day and night, (withdrawing from everything else), and concentrates on making his fortune. A time comes, when all the hard work and good luck merge together, (Emptiness) and the businessman attains what he wan ts. (Clarity). This could happen for the artist who wishes fame and glory. His talent and relentless effort, together with his connections, result in little waste of time before he attains these goals. Satisfied and full of joy, there is nothing more to wish for until he finds another venture.

We get caught up in the circle of pain and pleasure, poverty and riches, sickness and health, winning and losing... in short, the dualities of life. However, a meditator/orasyones balances his needs, fulfilling his responsibility to himself and to society at the same time, directing his efforts to the attainment of clarity and deeper understanding in the spiritual and intuitive spheres of life.

Self-actualization and clarity on the spiritual level are permanent and provide a balance as we grow in life. This is the highest form of self-fulfillment. We can call this the stage of Enlightenment or Clarity of Self.

This is the stage of Martial Art Mastery... The Way of Peace.

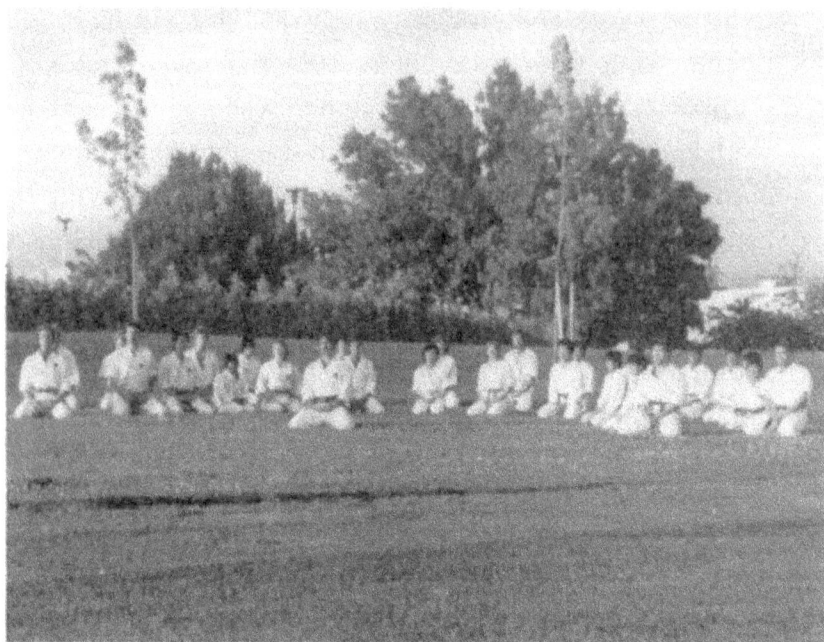

X.

TIPS FOR MEDITATORS/ ORASYONES

1) It is best to have a personal teacher. I will refer to this point in a further section.

2) It is best to empty your stomach 20 to 30 minutes before Dasal or meditating. Getting rid of poisons by fasting once in a while is also beneficial. Avoiding red meat and maintaining a light diet is suggested for the advanced meditator/orasyones.

3) The best times for meditation/Dasal are during sunrise and sunset, (or twice each day). If you have more time, you can perform Dasal at noon and at midnight, (or four times each day).

4) A half-bath neutralizes the temperature of your body. Wash your face wit h cool water. Wash the back of your neck and ears and rinse your mouth. Wash your hands from elbows down to the palms. Wash your

legs from knees to toes. Do this every time, prior to meditation/ Dasal, except when you take a full bath. This practice helps you awaken your energy center s and prepares you for deep meditation and orasyon.

5) Choose a spot in your room for meditation, thinking of it as an alter. If you have a spar e room, use it for meditation and health exercises. Face the East. This practice helps you to focus your entire energy on meditation/Dasal. It is important to have consistency and stability in your practice. Using one spot consistently and facing in a given direction, put your mind and your energy into focus.

6) Burn incense in the room.

7) Hang only photos or posters that are calming and relaxing to your mind.

8) You may play meditation music, chant or sing relaxing or devotional songs. This helps you to withdraw from outside distractions and to release tension from your system. Music and other sounds are more powerful forms of mental attractions.

9) Movement centering: Kiirtan/Ati-Atihan. While you are singing or chanting mantras and Dasal, (i.e. Babanam Kevalam), move your body around in a free movement, clap your hands, move your head about, all according to the tone of the chant. Later,

you might stand and dance, bending your knees in every step, touching the back of your left heel with the toes of your right foot, spreading both arms, projecting upwards in a Palm Salutation by placing both palms together and resting them at the center of your chest.

You may beat drums or play musical instruments. Chant and dance for 10 to 15 minutes. This is a form of active meditation, helping you to center yourself. It releases tension, calms the mind for better concentration and also subdues the ego.

10) Sit and meditate/Dasal. Beginners should try to practice for 20 to 30 minutes, while advanced students should devote from 45 minutes to one hour to meditation/Dasal. Maintain a consistent length of time. It is better to meditate 30 minutes twice daily than 2 hours every second day.

11) Lead a clean, moderate lifestyle.

12) Maintain an open mind and continuously grow and share.

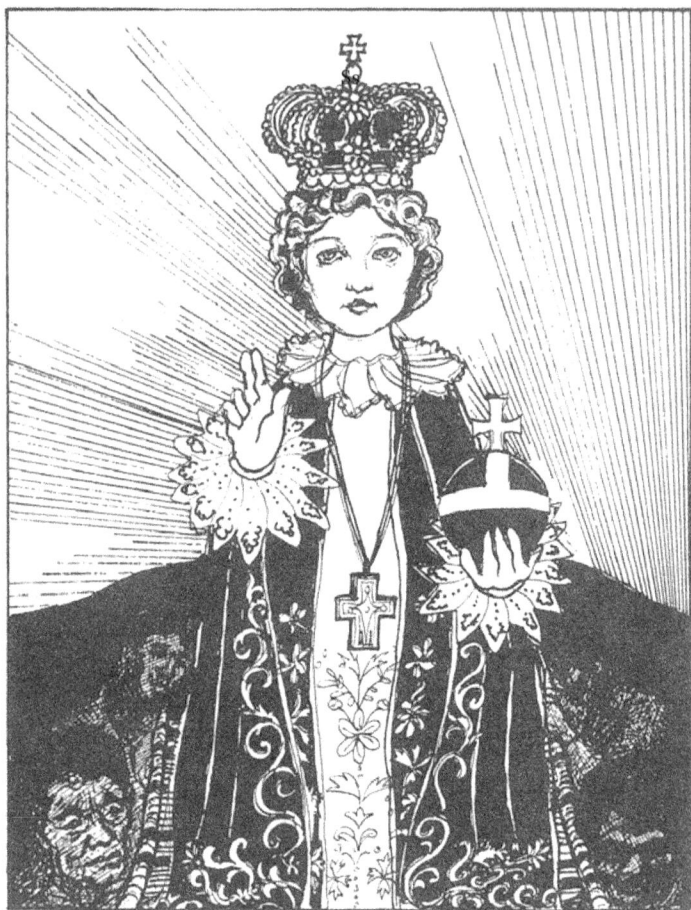

Santo Ninyo

XI

MEDITATIVE STRETCHING EXERCISES

Stretching exercises are non-extraneous. This is a complete form of health discipline directed toward the internal organs in our body, releasing both energy blocks and bodily tensions, maintaining the flow of circulation, massaging both muscles and nerves and twisting and stretching the joints and skeletal system. This is done through *relaxation, deep breathing, twisting and stretching with mental ease.* Stretching is the basis of ALL "warm-ups" and general exercises.

There are hundreds of exercise postures. Adopting a few of them and practicing these regularly is the key to mastery and health.

Simple Meditative and Dasal Exercises

1) Neck rotation   4) Body Rotation

2) Shoulder rotation   5) Leg Stretch

3) Body Twist   6) Deep Breathing
                                (found on page 52)

Choose to do your exercises before or after meditation/ Dasal. It is best to practice the same pattern of exercises to derive the maximum results.

WARM-UPS – EXERCISES

1) Neck Rotation (standing)

2) Shoulder Rotation (standing)

3) Hip Stretch, left and right,

4) Back Stretch, backward and forward

5) Knee & Ankle Rotation

6) Dancer's Pose

7) Balance pose

8) Squat Pose

This is the spiritual Essence of "Kata". Forms in Martial Arts, dance-like movements of punching and kicking, etc., are symbols of a Warrior fighting to attain liberation.

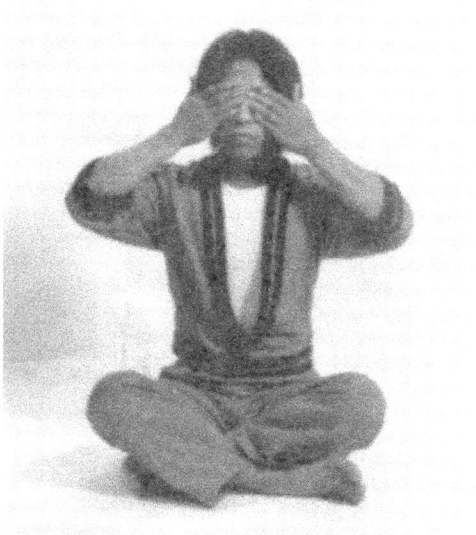

Fig 1-A Bow your head and raise it again, backward, 4 times.

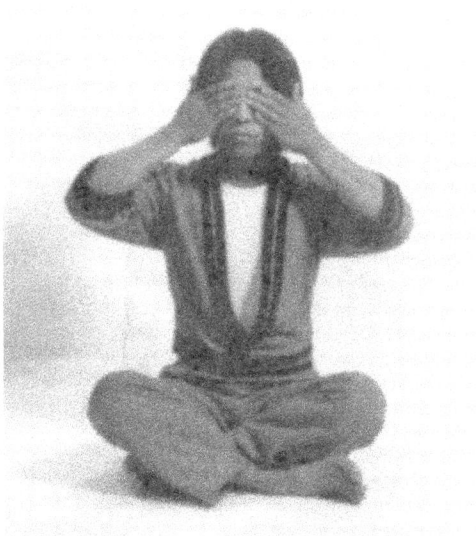

Fig 2-A Follow with careful, circular motions.

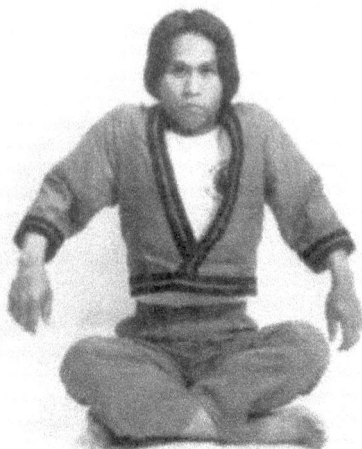

Fig 3-A Inhale as you raise shoulder.

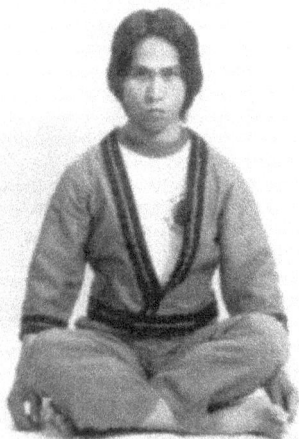

Fig 4-A Release shoulder tension as you exhale.

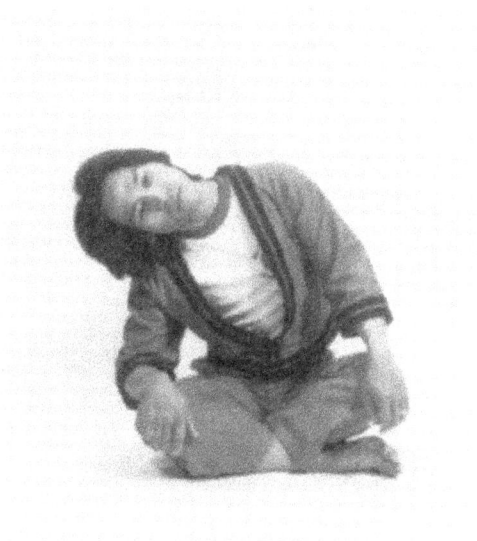

Fig 5-A Move head and body from side to side four times.

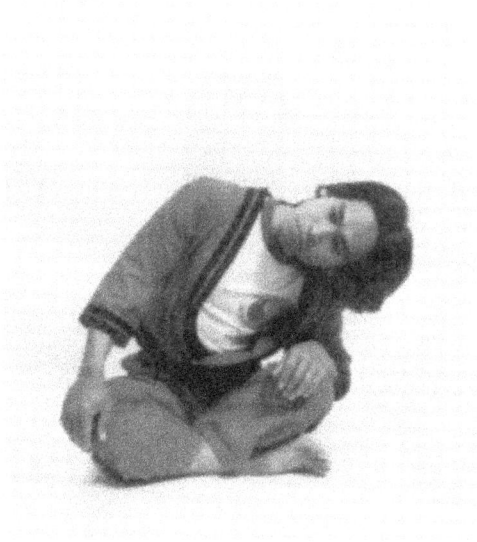

Fig 6-A Follow with careful circular motions.

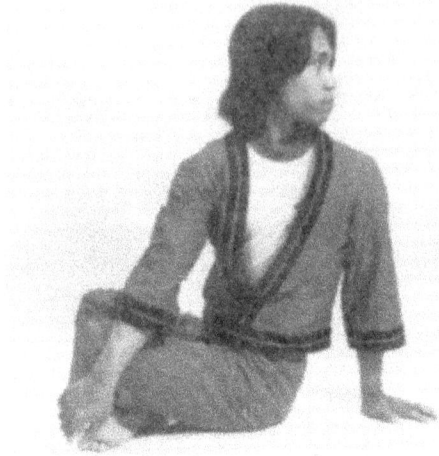

Fig 7-A Twist spine fully. Look behind you.

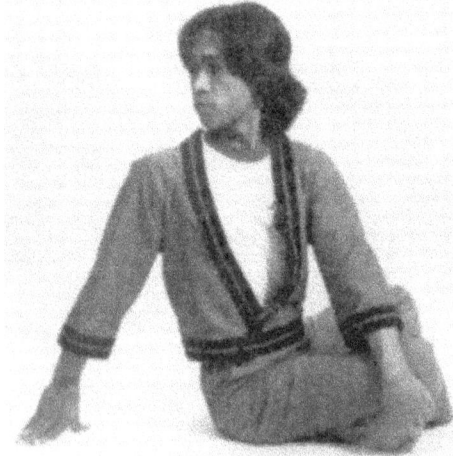

Fig 8-A Reverse the twist slowly, carefully.

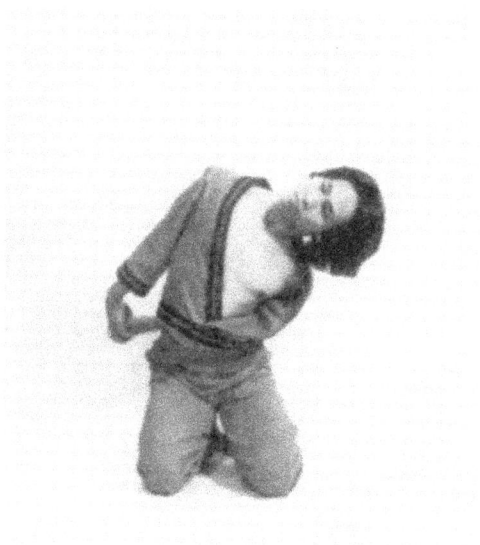

Fig 9-A Clasp hands behind you and bend sideways. Return.

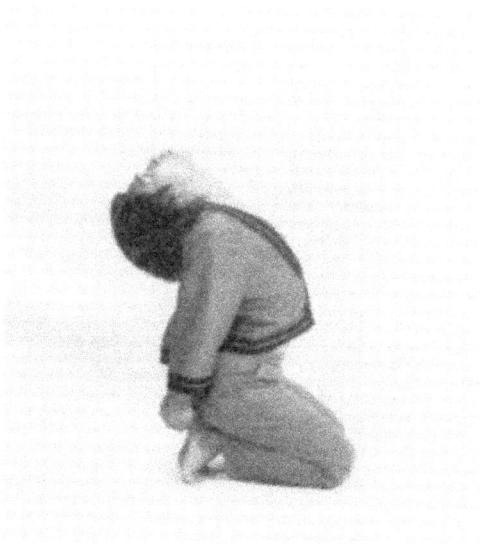

Fig 10-A Now bend slowly backwards and return.

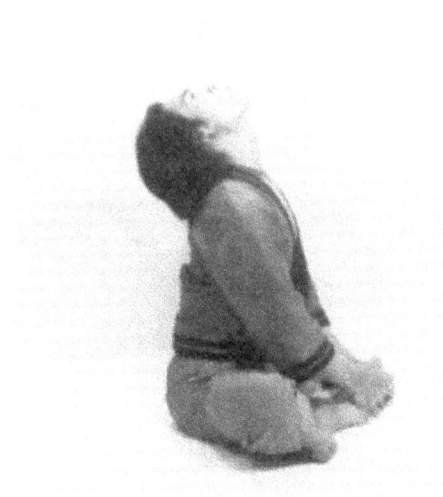

Fig 11-A Bring feet together and inhale as head is raised back.
Inhale fully.

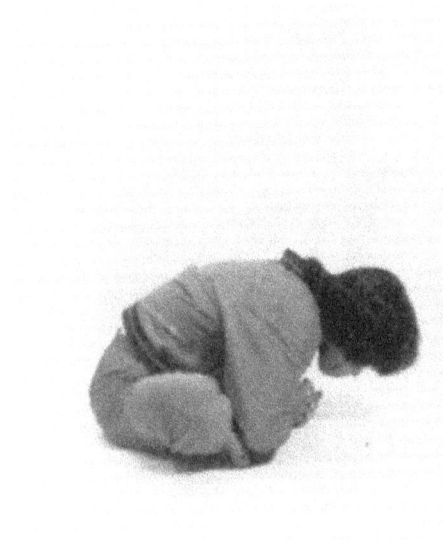

Fig 12-A Bend forward as you exhale.

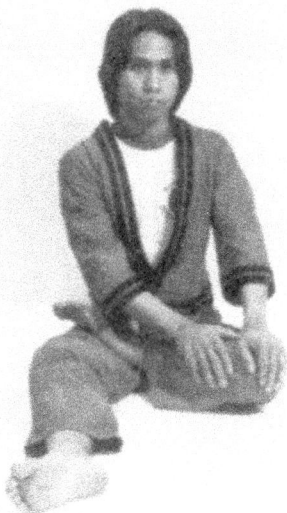

Fig 13-A Place right foot over left out stretched leg.

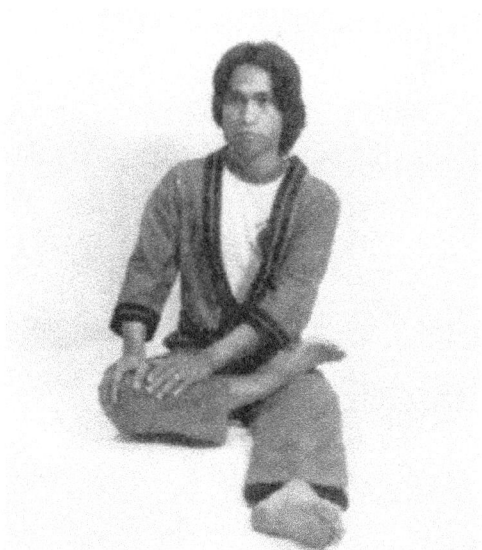

Fig 14-A Press down on bent knee. Now change legs.

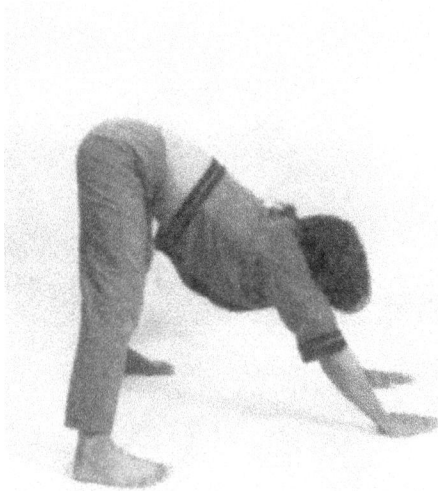

Fig 15-A With feet apart, place hands flat on floor ahead of you.

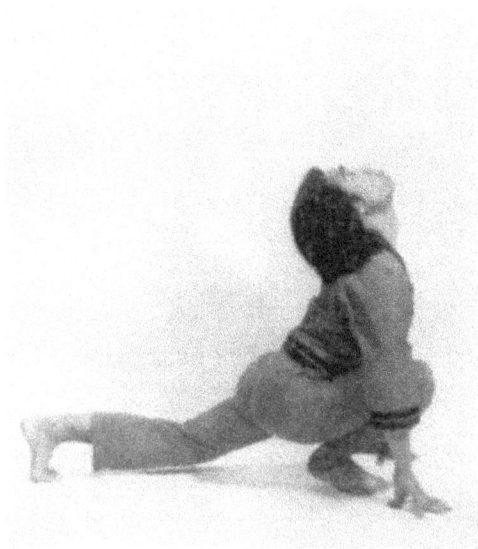

Fig 16-A Stoop down and place left foot back.
Bend head gently backward. Change legs.

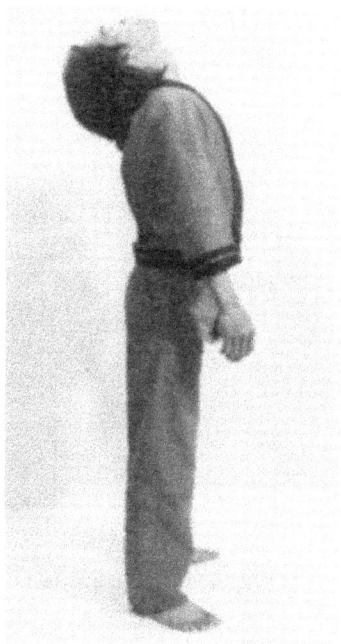

Fig 17-A
Feet apart, make a slow
circular motion of the head...

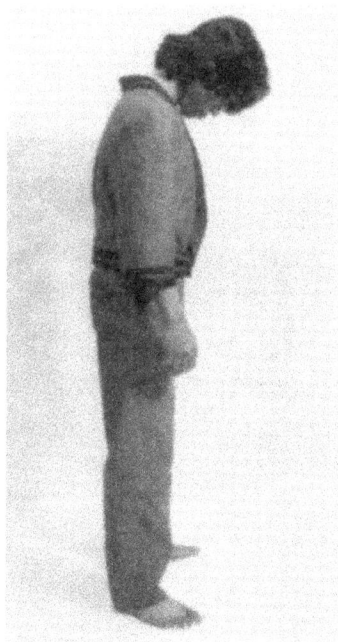

Fig 18-A
...fully and care fully.

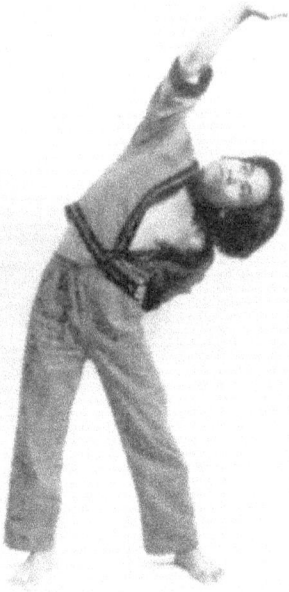

Fig 19-A Hand high, feet wide apart, stretch to the left.

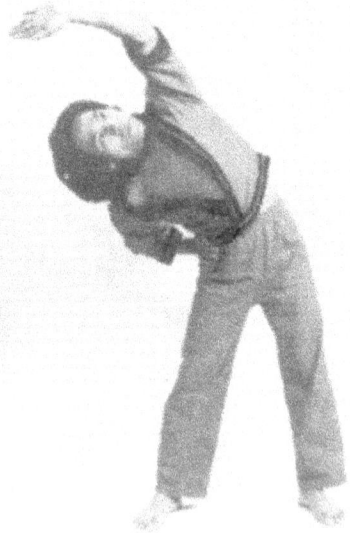

Fig 20-A Stretch right, using same posture.

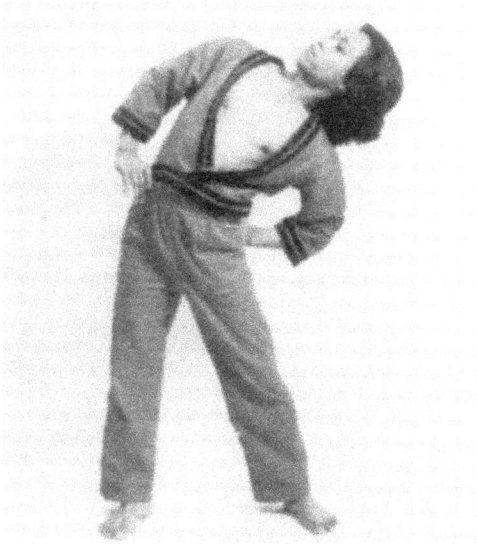

Fig 21-A Make a full circular motion, as you stretch backward.

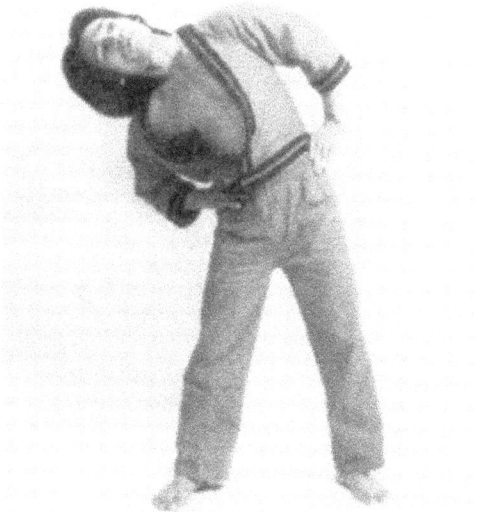

Fig 22-A Keep feet apart, exhaling on the return.

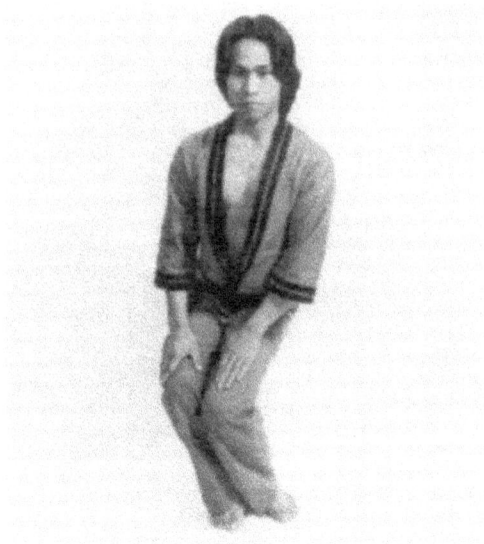

Fig 23-A Bend your knees and move them in a full circle. Always fully.

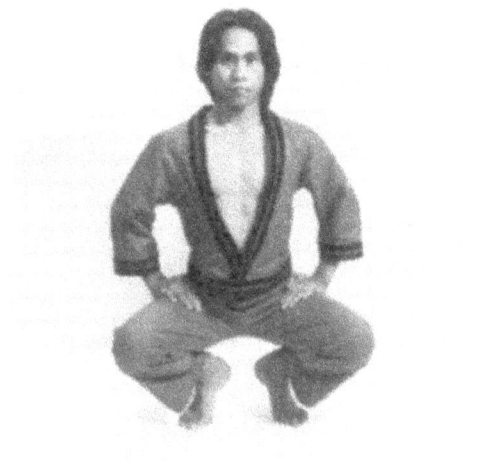

Fig 24-A Keeping knees straight,
bend down and place hands on knees.

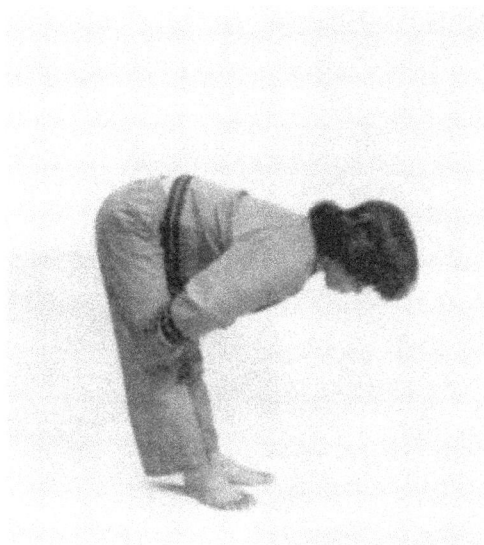

Fig 25-A Bend knees to squat position, hands on thighs.

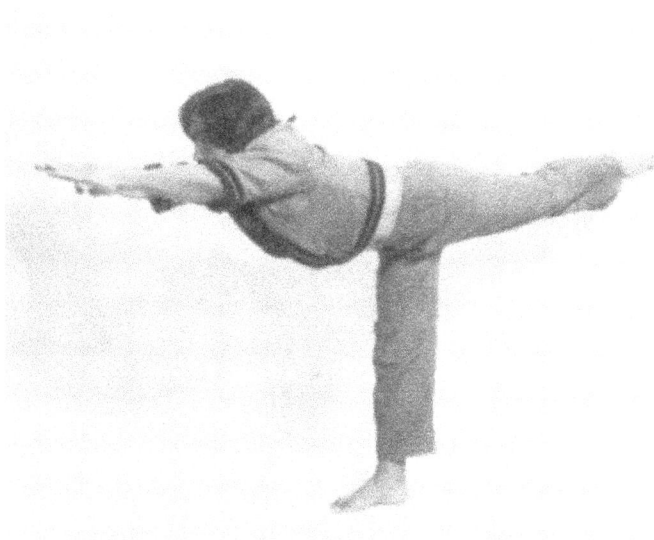

Fig 26-A Balance body on left foot, arms out stretched. Change feet.

81

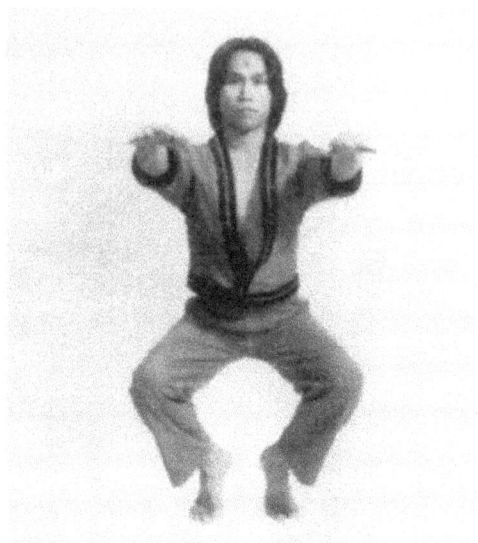

Fig 27-A With arms forward, bend knees to half squat.

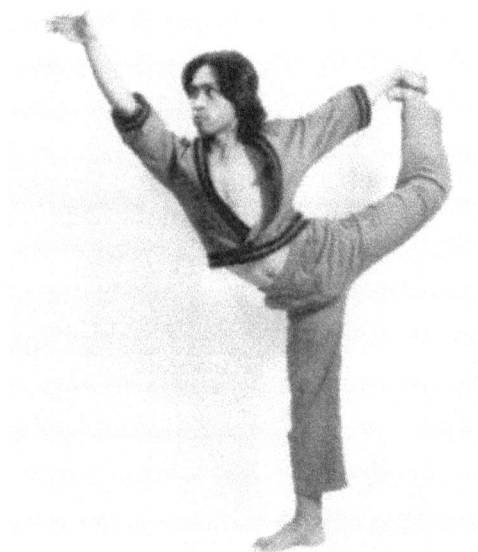

Fig 28-A While standing on right foot, take hold of left foot from the back. Repeat, changing feet.

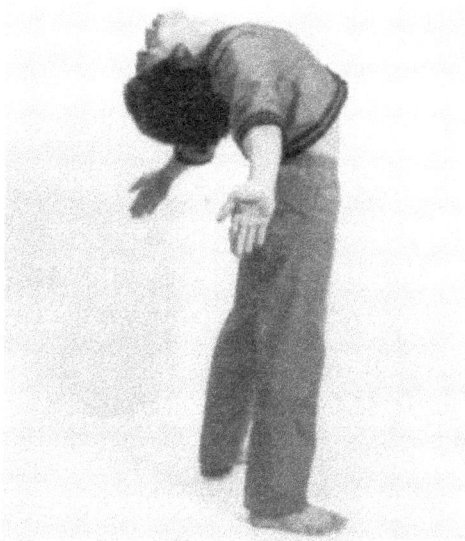

Fig 29-A Bend slowly backward, feet apart. Inhale as you go back. Return exhale.

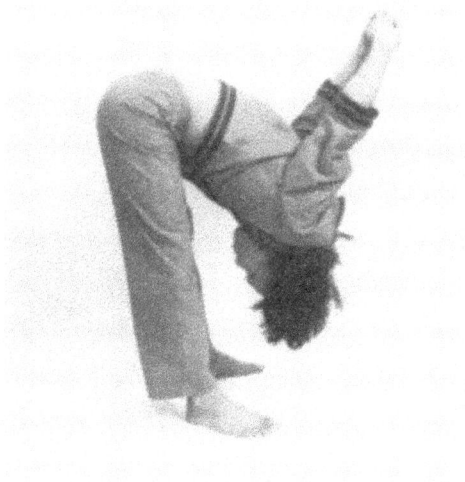

Fig 30-A Return while exhaling, until you are bent forward.

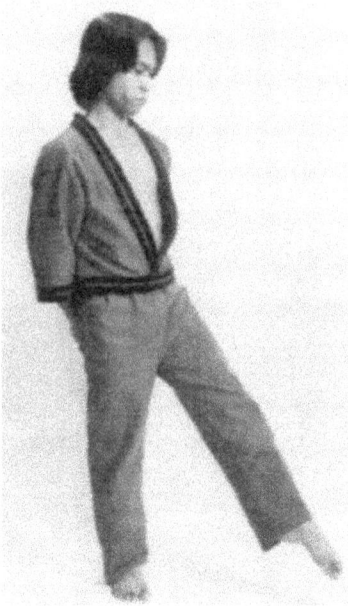

Fig 32-A Now move toes upward and down ward, followed by slow circles.

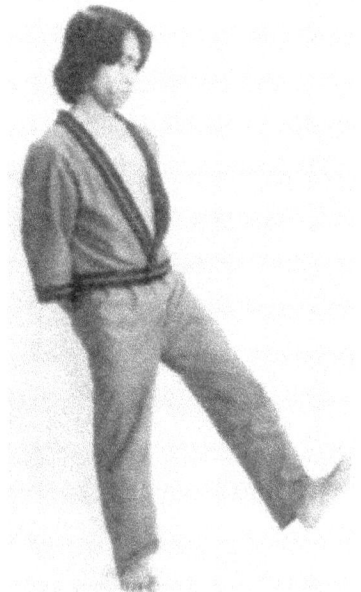

Fig 31-A Straighten toes as you lift leg forward.

XII.

MASSAGE – MASAHE
– AN "INWARD EXERCISE"

Following exercise, it is important to bring back to the body, a balance, a quietening or relaxation.

Any one form of exercise cannot give the body a complete and deep workout. There are always certain areas of the body that will be unmoved or unaffected. For example, Martial Arts does not affect certain areas of the bod y, such as back of the ear, armpit or nerve centers in the body, generally.

Asanas and Stretching exercises are forms of bodily massage, due to their twisting and pulling motion. The various bodily postures also regulate the harmony among external and internal muscles. After Asanas, carry out self-massage, Hilot and Masahe, using your fingers with gentle pressure in a twisting rotation of the palms and fingertips. Include your head, face, back of neck, shoulders, arms, chest, abdomen, back, thighs, legs and feet in your massage routine. In doing this, you will release the necessary energy flow throughout the body.

Self-massage and Masahe have many benefits. For example, massaging the abdomen, while coordinating our breathing, helps greatly to relieve tensions in the area. Experience the total relaxation this creates. Self-massage and Masahe after exercise are important, because they give us an opportunity to communicate with our own physical being, through the sense of touch. Even though we wash our body as a daily habit, we tend to lose touch with our physical selves. Sometimes, in spite of our body's aches and pains, we numb our feelings in order that we can continue to socialize and carry on our working day. Often, we will fail to pay attention to our body's complaints, until we are almost crippled or ill. At that point, we expect our physician to quickly remedy our problems. However, if we take care of ourselves on a daily basis, hopefully including massage and Masahe, our relaxation may result in less physical harm to our body from the wear of tensions. It is a joy to live in a healthy body! Naturally, we will quickly seek guidance from our physician, if pain and feelings of illness continue to affect our well-being.

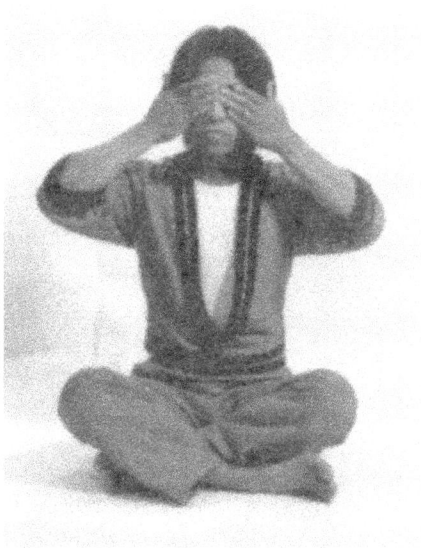

Fig 1-B Gently press your eyes with the tips of your fingers.

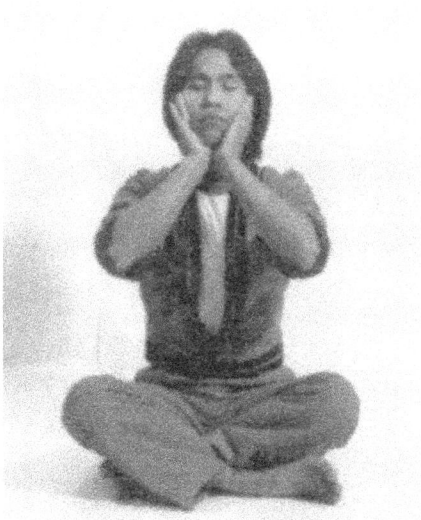

Fig 2-B Press beneath jaw with thumbs, palms against face.

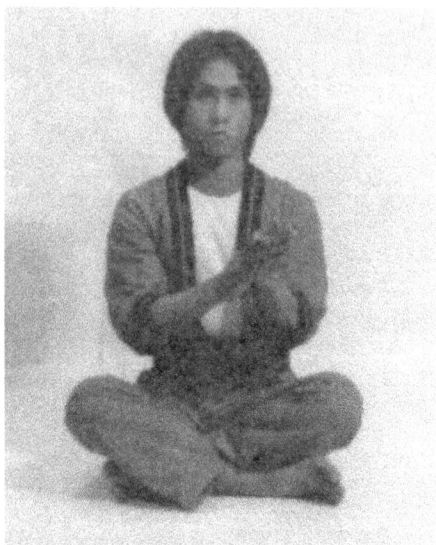

Fig 3-B Rub both palms together, while sitting cross legged.

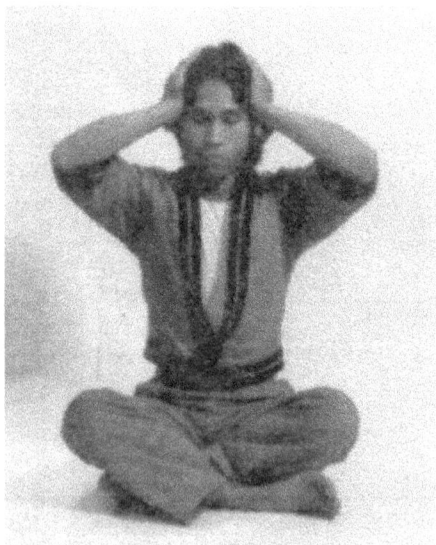

Fig 4-B Press both the temples with the palms.

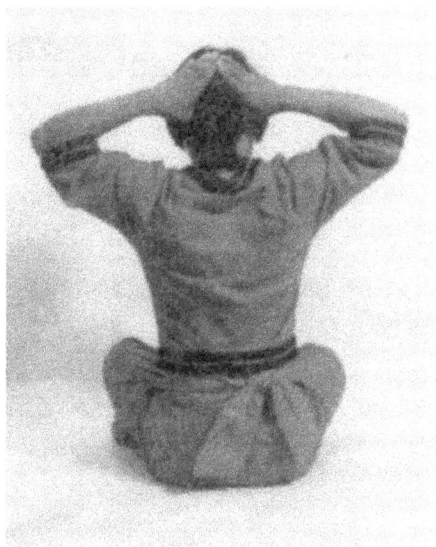

Fig 5-B Massage the shoulders with the fingertips.

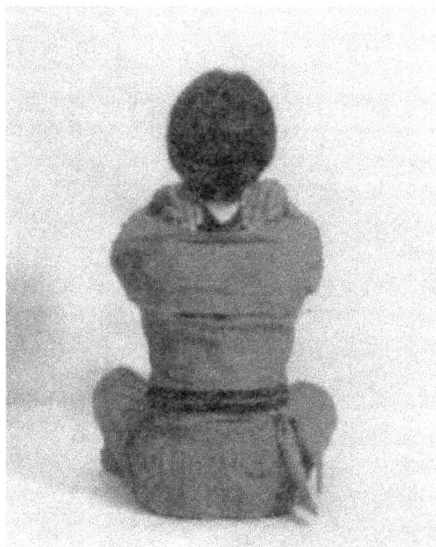

Fig 6-B Press back neck with both thumbs.

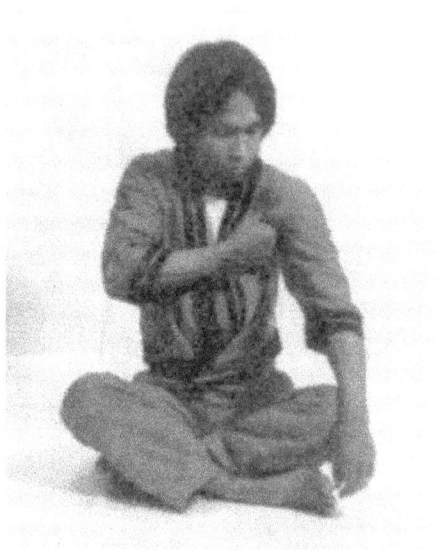

Fig 7-B Massage your right armpit with left hand, then left armpit, etc.

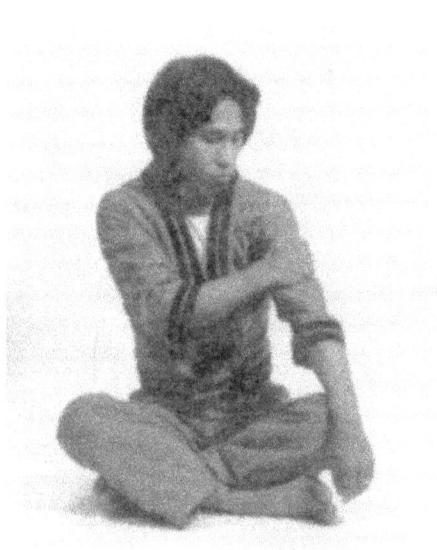

Fig 8-B Massage upper arm with your left hand and change sides, etc.

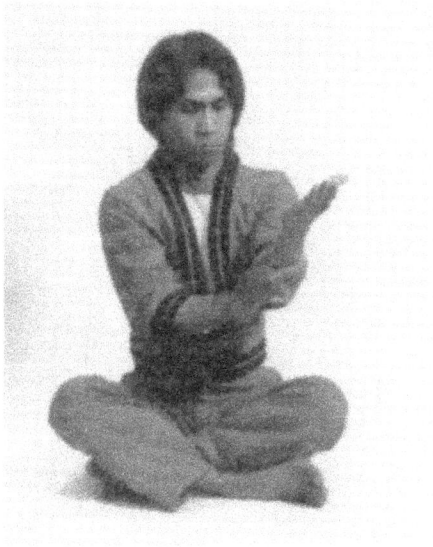

Fig 9-B Massage forearm with thumbs and fingertips.

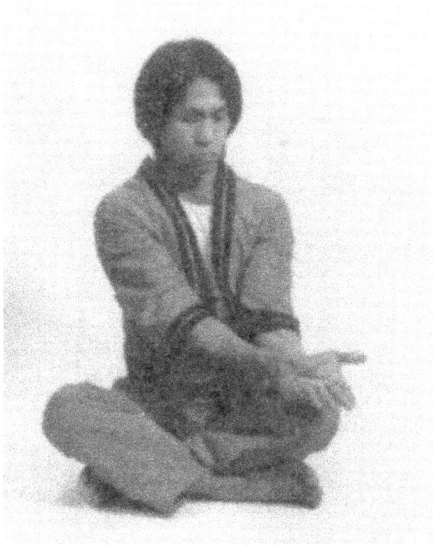

Fig 10-B Press your palm deeply with the thumb.

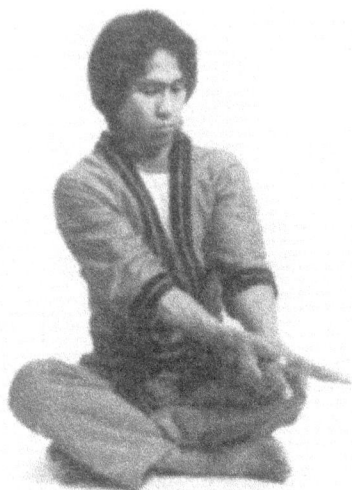

Fig 11-B Press the back of your hand with your thumb.

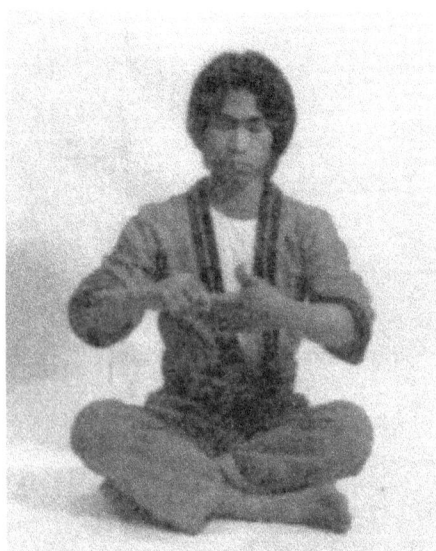

Fig 12-B Knead each finger with the opposite fingers.

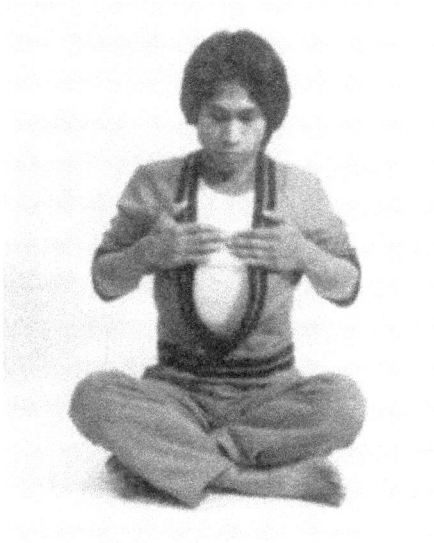

Fig 13-B Press the breastbone with palms and spread fingers.

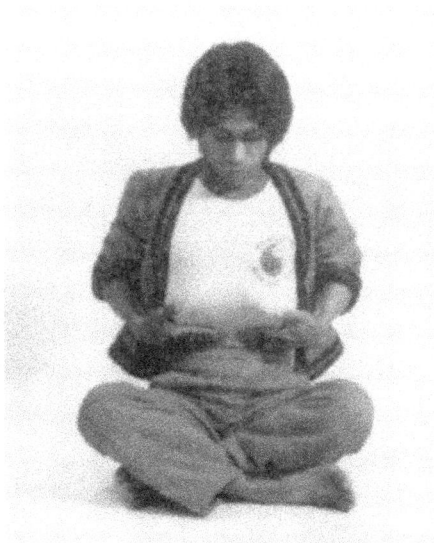

Fig 14-B Press diaphragm with all fingers.

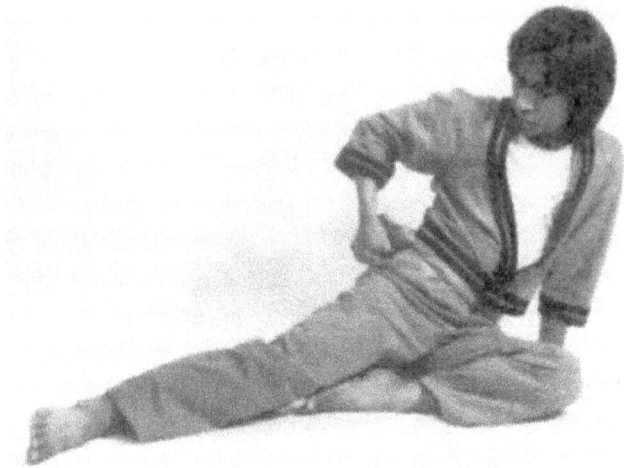

Fig 15-b Sitting with one leg extended, knead the sides of that hip with your thumbs. Change to opposite side.

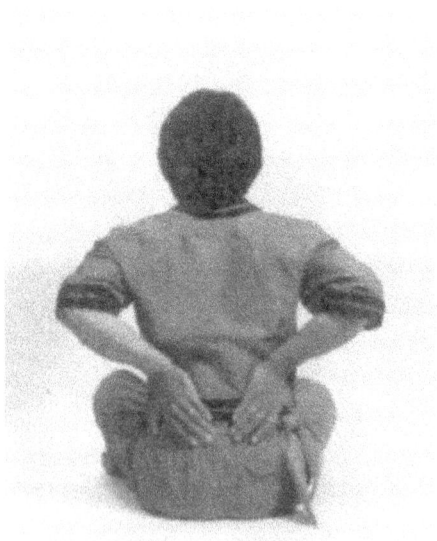

Fig 16-B Press your lower back with your palms.

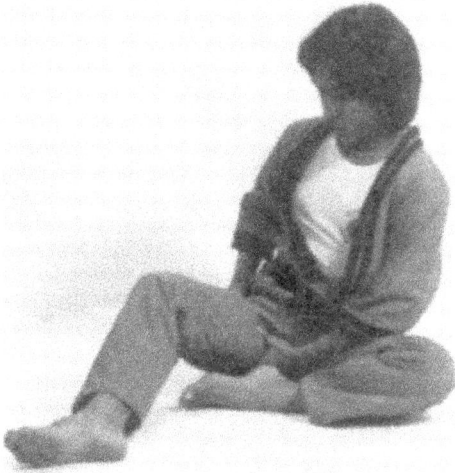

Fig 17-B Circle hands abound upper thigh and knead muscles.

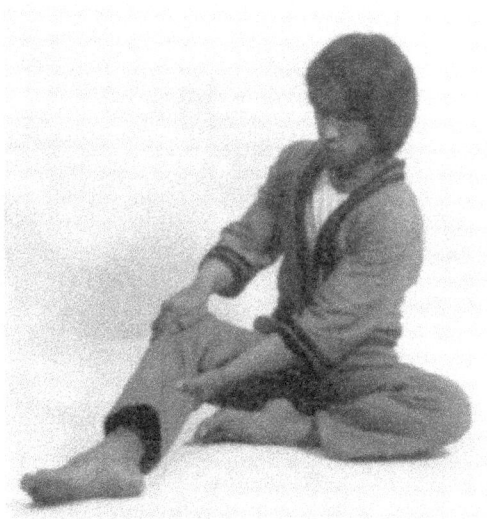

Fig 18-B Massage calf muscles down to ankle.

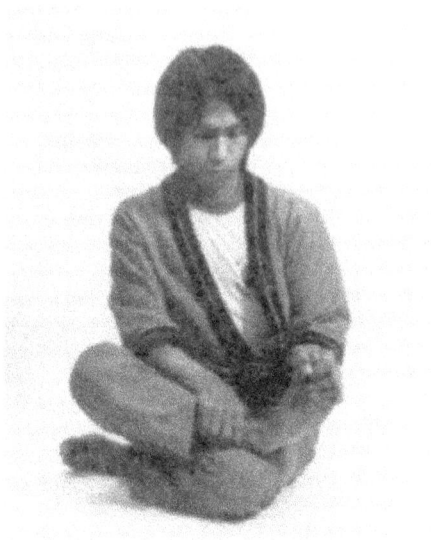

Fig 19-B Knead the upper foot with the thumbs.

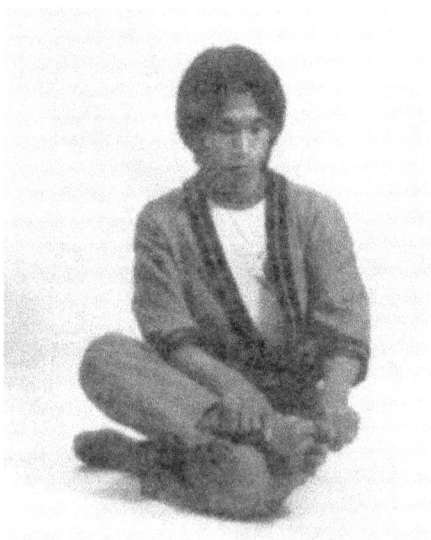

Fig 20-B Knead tendons of the ankle with the thumbs.

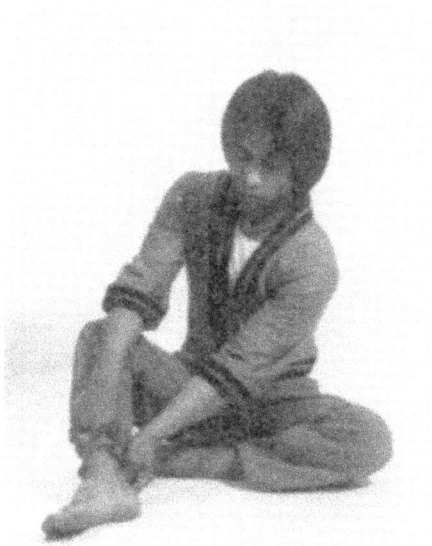

Fig 21-B Rotate ankle fully in each direction.

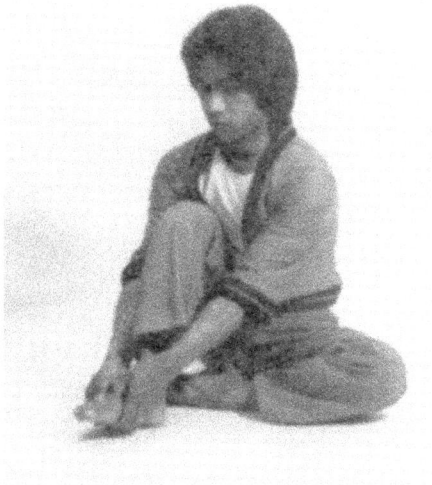

Fig 22-B With the legs crossed, knead each toe.

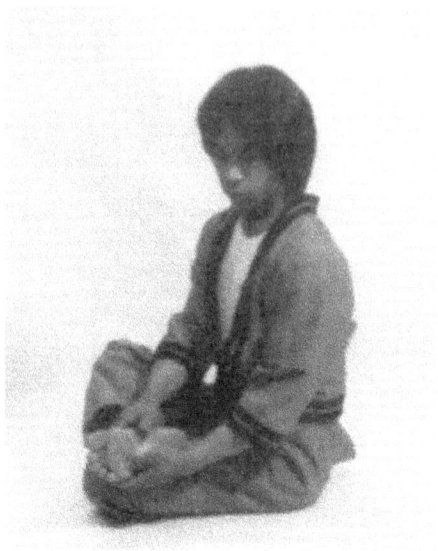

Fig 23-B Gently massage the sole of the foot with your thumb

XIII

INWARD EXERCISE-FLOW

LAKAS – ENERGY FLOW...
MEDITATION/ORASYON IN ACTION

There will always be similarities in different forms of exercises and flexibility techniques. No matter how complicated the differences, (dependent upon the system or teacher), similarities will exist. This is also true in the case of all human beings, born to live in a complicated world, using complicated life styles, until they depart in their own time.

In everything, there is always a beginning or base. There is a process and a goal. We cannot function without either a base or purpose.

The same theory is reflected in the different training exercises and in Martial Arts. Regardless of any differences in technique, there is always the same base and goal. For example, I have observed that all Martial Arts and sport sessions begin with a warm-up; relaxation, loosening and stretching exercises. The difference comes in the techniques used. Some favor more hand techniques, others, the feet, either using the body for shifting and leaping, or moving in a straight or circular motion, etc. Again, it will depend upon the founder of the exercises or techniques. However, we will notice that all forms and techniques lead to mental relaxation, release of energy, body fitness, self-confidence, etc. These become the goal.

The most common source of good, one which we normally take for granted, is the energy flow, known in the Orient as the Lakas Khi, Chi, Prana or vital force.

Whether it is internal or external force, we always use strength or power-energy flow. The difference is noticed, and may vary, according to the energy level of each individual. Naturally, th ere are different forms of energy waves or vibrations. It will depend upon the degree of personal power.

- Internal Energy
- Spiritual Force
- Subtle Force
- Cosmic Power
- Universal Energy
- Unlimited Energy
- Infinite Force.

It is very difficult to conceptualize Lakas, Prana or internal energy in any form of rational understanding. Lakas is beyond boundaries; it can only be experienced and realized.

It is only through releasing energy block s, going th rough a cleansing process and maintaining purity of mind and body, that we will experience the unlimited source of energy we call "Lakas".

Knowingly or unknowingly, we are always in touch with our Lakas force. This energy gives us all the strength we need to achieve pro per direction in our day-to-day life. It is expressed at all levels of motion. We have heard of people who have lifted heavy weights or who have run f aster than anybody could imagine, while under extreme threat or pressure.

Lakas can also be seen in the Martial Artist who executes a feat without using any apparent physical force. Internal energy allows the Martial Artist to perform super-human acts, such as breaking bricks, jumping to great heights, leaping like a cat, making the body either heavy or light or being able to attain whatever is projected in the mind. Lakas internal Force is evidenced in being able to heal, attain fulfillment and peace of mind.

We saw Terry Fox on his run across Canada, in his effort to enlighten the consciousness of others and to raise funds for the Cancer Society. A feat of such proportions by this handicapped man demonstrates an outstanding Lakas. Bruce Lee, who in his lifetime, became the most famous Oriental person in the world, also relied on Lakas for his accomplishments. Using his internal energy, he portrayed so vividly, the image of the Martial Artist.

Great men and women who have tapped their potentials and succeeded in their quests as hum an beings, great personalities who have broken out of the traditional ways to become the true pioneers in society these people are examples of those who have dared to go beyond the usual limits to become the seers of a new understanding. Gurus, saints, personalities known and unknown, have all attained th rough their Lakas energy, their source of in finite power. With the Lakas energy, we can attain the ultimate understanding of the universe.

NEGATIVE LAKAS ENERGY – MISDIRECTED FORCE – EGO POWER

Lakas, Chi, Pran a or Internal (vital) Force, like everything else, has a negative side. This means that a person who attains a certain amount of Lakas can be destructive, due to a personal ego "trip", the desire for fame and power, for instance.

Here, the Lakas energy turns into a psychic force. It becomes a complete concentration of mind. When engrossed in fulfilling one's personal desires, these energies can be called:

- Corrupt
- Mean
- Black Magic
- Witchcraft
- Evil
- Power Hungry

Unfortunately, these particular forces are easier to attain. This involves only complete discipline of mind, projection of one's thoughts and complete concentration of one's individual energy into one's self-centered desire. An example would be an egocentric individual willing to sacrifice everything of value to reach a certain goal.

Such energy can direct the mind along one path, without necessarily following any principles or moral ethics. We have seen a great number of people at these negative levels of energy. From politicians, military experts, "sports" people all the way down to street hustle rs, we see them all, power-hungry directed energies.

Naturally, when we miss the right direction or path, we are lost. The more blind we become, the more we tend to err. The more often we bang our heads against a brick wall, the more it hurts! Each time it hurts, it indicates that there is a block. At this point, we can either "clean up our act", purify ourselves and begin in a new path, directing our force with a pos1t1ve image or the Lakas energy will destroy us.

There is only one source of Lakas or power; that is the total Energy of the Universe. The cosmic energies are pure and subtle. We cannot have these energies, if we are crudely made of "blocks."

We can only have the Lakas energy if we open our mind and body, and listen to the flow of nature.

As my Master said, "You are never alone. The Force that guides the stars, guides you also."

The following illustrations, Fig. 33, 34 and 35, demonstrate moments in the continuous movement of the **bracing** exercise.

In rhythm with your breathing

a) Raise arms overhead, while inhaling and exhale a you lower them slowly downward.

b) Repeat this in a circular motion, coordinating breathing with movement.

c) Relax at all times throughout the exercise.

d) Maintain a feeling of force coming from the abdomen.

e) When exhaling, feel the force releasing th rough the palms.

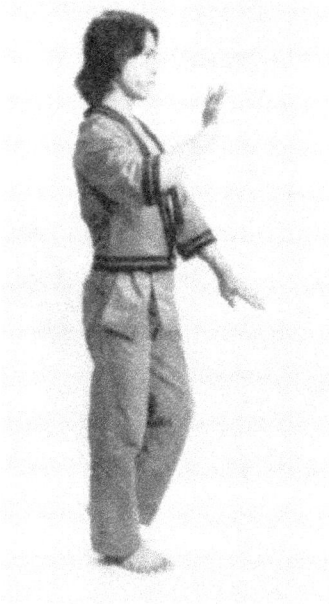

Fig 33 Up Left

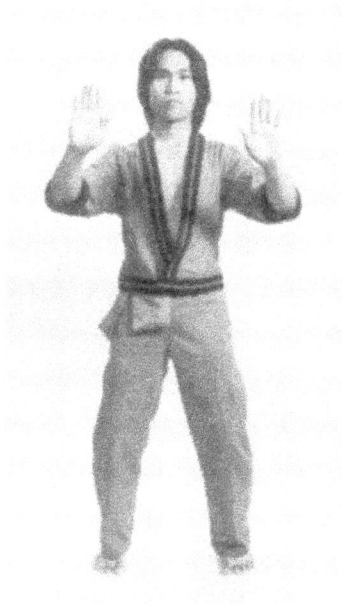

Fig 34 Up Right

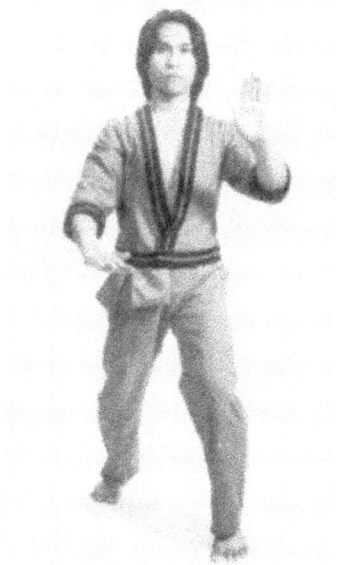

Fig 35 Right

XIV

CORPSE POSITION

It is important to mentally relax the entire system. This relaxation technique is called the Corpse Position.

This relaxation technique is called the Corpse Position.

Lie flat on your back, spreading your legs apart. Spread both arms to the sides of your body, palms upward. Close your eyes. Slowly move all the parts of your body to relax them. Think deeply, feeling the relaxation, part by part. First, concentrate on the right leg. Inhale, and slowly raise that leg, tens e it fully and hold your breath. After a few seconds, exhale quickly and relax the muscles of your right leg, letting it fall to the floor on its own, without using any force. Then, slowly find the most comfortable position for your right leg, by either shaking it or moving it into its proper place.

Repeat the same procedure, using your left leg, and then both hands, one at a time.

Now, concentrate fully on the muscles of the pelvis, buttocks and abdominal area. Once again, tense and relax the muscles. Inhale deeply through your nose, extending both abdomen and chest area, and then exhale completely, ridding yourself of all energy blocks or tensions. Through relaxed breathing, inhale and feel a warm energy fully comforting your entire system. Exhale and feel the tension releasing as if through your nose.

This is complete relaxation; even your mind is at rest now. Notice how easily your breath flow s in and out. Notice the thoughts running through your mind without force or pressure. You may feel as if you are witnessing yourself from afar.

Stay still for a few minutes. When you decide to "awaken" from this relaxed state, imagine the refreshed energy flowing into each part of your body, beginning with your head and moving downward, all the way to your toes. You will slowly move the different parts of your body, while taking a deep breath. Bring both feet together, moving them to the left or to the right. Bring your hands up over your head. Slowly stretch, like a cat does, before he fully awakens. Now, turn to your right side and gently sit up for meditation and Dasal.

The benefits will be quickly apparent to you. Your body will be totally relaxed. Practice the corpse pose when you are exhausted or before Orasyon. This important relaxation method can be practiced anytime, in almost any place you may happen to be, if the environment is suitable, (as I have outlined in previous pages).

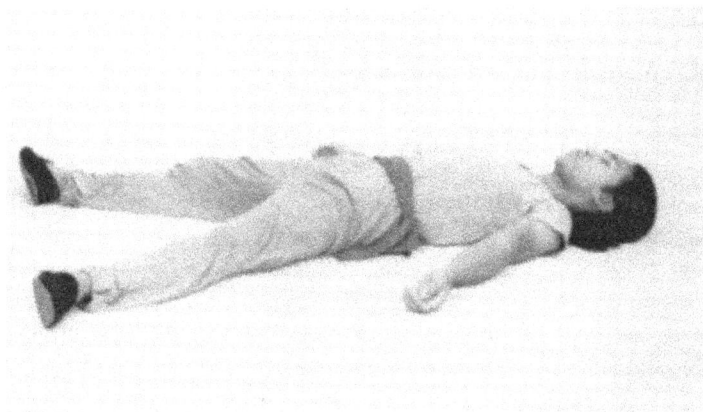

Fig 6 The full Corpse Position, a moment of total relaxation.

XV

DIET

There are three levels of practitioner. The first one is the person who practices self- discipline techniques for physical conditioning. The second one is the person who practices techniques for both mental relaxation and physical health. The third person is one w ho carries out both exercises and Meditation/Dasal, and also practices its teachings and way of life at the same time.

It is important for the advanced practitioner to have a wholesome and health y diet. Over the years, practitioners have come to value these guidelines:

We will consider three categories of foods:

STATIC – not good for the body and possibly, the mind; liquor, strong spirits, drugs, synthetic and chemically-derived foods, indulgence in red meat.

MUTATIVE – foods of doubtful value; over-cooked foods of all kinds, candies, chocolate, chemically preserved and dehydrated products, coffee, over-ripe foods, over-indulgence in white meat and eggs.

SENTIENT – good for total health; green, fresh vegetables; milk and dairy products, fruits and nuts, grains, soy products, herbs, honey, (clean fresh drinking and cooking water).

NOTE: Although not a food, cigarettes are considered Static, with no value to the body or mind, whatsoever.

It ha s been recorded in scientific literature that a vegetarian diet is preferred to that of a regime high in meat products. Let it be said that a good balance in food intake is important for the health of body and mind.

XVI.

FASTING

Fasting is one of the most useful cleansing processes to purify both our body and mind. It has been said that it is best to fast during the full moon or new moon, for the sun and the moon exert gravitational pull, causing the liquid and gaseous factors in the body to rise up, obstructing our chest and mind, causing a disturbing feeling. Fasting empties the digestive tract and helps to counteract this imbalance.

Fasting also removes accumulated toxins and gives some rest to the body. If you feel strong, attempt a full fast, 24 hours, from sunrise to sunrise. Break your fast gently, taking lemon water at first, then fruits, followed by a meal. You can also carry out liquid fasting or "half fasting". During fasting, you should perform more mental and spiritual work, trying not to exert yourself physically.

It is to be remembered that we are already experienced in fasting, going each day, twelve hours without food, from six p.m. to six a.m., with our first meal called "breaking the fast" or breakfast.

XVII

DIFFERENT PATHS TO ENLIGHTENMENT

In ancient history, there were evolutionary social cycles. According to my Master, there once were four classes of people:

1) Sudra – (workers)

These were people whose main goal was to labor only in order to eat. They were usually content to be servants and laborers. Although they were strong workers, they required constant supervision. Throughout ancient times to the present day, society has erred in the use of these people in slavery.

2) Ksattriya – (Warriors)

The warriors had a strong sense of loyalty, determination, and were good soldiers. They carried a powerful belief in their masters and in their service under him. The social cycle in this period saw people governed through a militant state.

3) Vipra – (Intellectuals)

These were creative people, ingenious as philosophers and preachers. They had strong mental abilities that made them superior thinkers, but they were weak in the roles of laborer and warrior.

4) Vaeshya – (Merchants)

The Vaeshya were skilled in the art of manufacturing products and making profits. They capitalized on the qualities of workers, warriors and intellectuals, and used the outcomes for their own purposes. These people had good organizational and managerial skills. The resulting social cycle, a trading one, followed the warrior era.

As we continued to develop our society, convenience was always the leading path toward progress. Each new invention reduced the necessity to labor, increasing the need for education, and, also, the competition for positions in society, however humble. Unfortunately, to succeed became increasingly difficult and continues in this pattern today. Guru Baba stresses the importance of the qualities in these four categories; hard worker, warrior, creator and organizer. These qualities, when combined, create a viksuda sudra, an *enlightened warrior.*

We all have, hidden within us, the qualities of the warrior. From the moment we are born, we struggle to survive. We study, we work, we love or hate in the effort to understand.

Life itself is a struggle, and, from the least of mankind to the highest position in our society, each one of us fights in order to reach our destiny. This is the reason why there are many ways or paths available to us to achieve our individual purpose. Paths Toward Enlightenment

1) The Path of Service (Karma) "Kabutihan"

    The worker who relies on good work and hard labor, and practices the path of service. In the Philippines, this practice is called Bayanihan. For example, the entire neighborhood volunteers when one villager is in need of help. Service is their way to enlightenment.

2) The Path of Intellect (Jhani) "Talino".

    The practitioner uses his creative works in order to expand and uplift his consciousness.

3) The Path of Love or Devotion. (Bhakti) "Pagmahal"

    The devotee gives nurturing and care to the needy. She practices devotion and selfless love to her path or master.

4) The Warrior's Path (Bushido) "Bayani".

    This is the path of discipline. The practitioner follows rigid discipline to strengthen himself, in order to serve and fight for justice.

How do we choose the right path? How do we choose a master who is right for us? For every problem, there is a solution, and with every solution, another obstacle appears. Problem solving itself is a path. It is the warrior's path. This truth means only that we have the solution for our problems and vice versa. This also means that *we are* the path to our destinies. We are the masters of our souls. This is the ultimate goal. This is *self-realization.*

Naturally, we all have to go through a life cycle of learning, from the moment we are born. I have watched my one year old son first make sound s, move his body, reach out. His busy hands, his large, curious eyes, every single part of his body reflects a constant awareness throughout the day. His whole being seemed to cry out, "I want to know, and I want to know now!"

Every child is a symbol of ourselves and our constant search for knowledge. We continuously learn from the time we are born, until the moment we pass away. We can certainly learn from our trials and errors, however, finding someone who truly understands life's patterns and who can guide us to the right path is much to be preferred.

I suggest that both approaches should be examined; first, learning through experience, and then, following a true teacher.

1) *Look Within* The student analyzes what he expects of himself, his own nature, his desires, his commitment. He analyzes whether or not the path he is choosing has advantages or disadvantages for his grow th.

2) *Outward Search* In this case, the student does not know what he wants. He requires external structures to follow. He must be willing to follow full instruction with complete devotion.

Each system has advantages and disadvantages. Searching within has a tendency to retain self-interest or "ego" that might prevent the student from making right decision s. At the same time, looking within and knowing what feels right and what does no t might assist him to chose the right path or teacher.

All students in the Outward Search must be aware of an ever present problem. The system of looking out ward makes the student vulnerable to exploitation and fanaticism. There is always the danger of not being able to think for oneself. We are all aware of many unscrupulous cults that have brought more harm than good to their followers!

The advantage of looking outward, provided the student finds the right teacher, is quicker growth toward maturity and peace, for he avoids much internal conflict. There is a total trust. There is no lingering doubt left in the mind of the student.

If you have some knowledge, follow the first system. Look within first, and th en choose the right path for yourself. Having done so, and you are not comfortable with your progress toward enlightenment, carefully choose a teacher whom you trust fully. Follow his instruction without getting side-tracked with your own personal knowledge. Always remember that you are a *student*.

If you do not have any knowledge about a path to follow, you might have to risk finding the right teacher for yourself. Start with someone you can get along with and trust. Check his background thoroughly and meet other people who have studied under him. Check him personally, finding out whether or not he is truly practicing what he is saying.

Once you find the teacher, follow him completely, learn everything that will help your growth, but do not accept inst ruction that you feel might hinder your progress. Choose only that which is helpful and stay away from that which is not.

There is a lot to be learned, a sea of knowledge, from the very smallest thing in creation to the wide universe. Each teacher and each path has something to offer. Each one attracts students according to their levels of consciousness. For instance, a warrior can relate more easily to a warrior's way. Likewise, we must all grow in our own way. We must change our perspective according to our grow th, as we do our teacher and our path. This does not mean that we must start all over again. On the contrary. We should allow these changes to permit goodness and maintain our very foundation.

As the son explores the world, he never forgets where he comes from. He uses more and more knowledge at different levels to strengthen his foundation. He gathers more strength from out side to balance his inner strength. Ultimately, this balance of internal and external is the *mastery*. This is the ultimate goal to find the master within us, to find our own path, to become enlightened.

"Seek and prepare, for when the time is right, the Master will come."

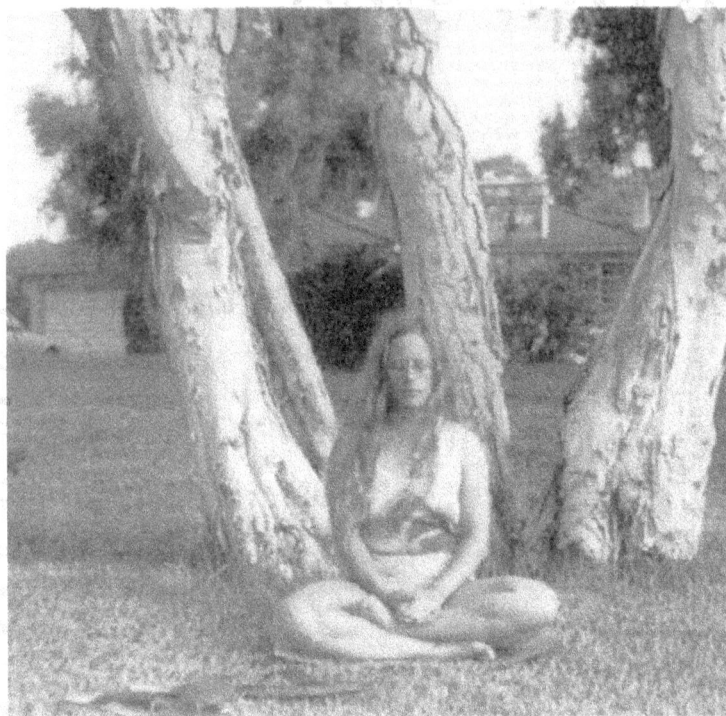

XVIII

WEAKNESSES

Each and everyone of us has weaknesses. However, our weaknesses can be our source of strength. Without weaknesses, there is no struggle, and without struggle, th ere is no life. There are two sides to weaknesses, the creative and the destructive. When we are weak, when we are down, sick or lost, the creative weakness, or positive attitude toward weakness, uses this stage to rest, to search, contemplate and purify. This stage of retreat is to accumulate the necessary strength to find solutions.

Destructive weakness is that which drives us into hopelessness, giving us a feeling of total helplessness. There is nothing to look forward to. There is no internal strength. There is only defeat. This is a very critical stage. If allowed to continue, it can mean failure to live effectively. But, for an enlightened warrior, defeat is a challenge to rise up again. He knows th a t the important rule is to do one's best in all situations.

This means that we cannot escape whatever we are doing. We cannot simply stop life stop ourselves from growing. We may delay or postpone our growth or maturing, but we cannot halt the natural progress of life. The fact that we are faced with a problem means that there is also a solution. Without problems, there would be no solution s, and vice versa. Therefore, weakness is only a temporary stage, a stage without answers. Although we all experience weaknesses, we need not despair. It is simply a matter of our preventing ourselves from getting caught up in the negative or the destructive side of our weaknesses.

We all pass through different stages of growing or understanding, whether during periods of weakness or strength, in ignorance or in knowledge, in situations either good or evil. These are all stages of growth. Every weakness that we overcome is a realization that we have acquired new strength. In the warrior's path, we are faced with constant difficulties, always a direct test of our own weaknesses and strengths. All the struggles and confusions we pass through are directed to ward facing ourselves. Ultimately, all our weaknesses, such as fear, doubt, anger, impatience, greediness, hate, lust or power challenge us to transform our failures into victories.

Every stage of growth presents to us many kind s of problems that bring out our weaknesses. We always eventually come face to face with our own weaknesses or failures. We have to accept these failures, and, somehow, direct them towards success and goodness. We cannot cut off the world or hide from ourselves. We can only transcend our weaknesses to live once again within our strengths. An individual in the warrior's path is faced with a constant struggle to keep himself at the level of strength. The warrior quickly recognizes his weaknesses and turns them into strength, without hesitation. This is a result of his being continuously on guard, never allowing himself to descend into the unhealthy depths of failure.

A Guru can be a more direct guide, preventing the student from falling prey to weakness. The teacher can have a strong impact on the student's self-discipline, until the student is able to develop an inner strength to take care of his own weaknesses.

Weaknesses are brought about by strong emotions, personal growth and an ever-wandering mind. With self-discipline, life encounters and know ledge, we can transform our weaknesses into strengths.

XIX.

ORASYON

Orasyon is a popular belief of the old folks in the Phil-ippines. It is said to be a system of magical prayers. The practitioners are in a deep trance when they repeat the orasyons. People who possess this power claim to be able to make them selves superhuman. From India we hear stories about yogi eating razor blades, drinking acid and sleeping on beds of nails. There are a few gurus who are said to be able to turn rocks into diamonds and heal sickness. From the realm of Japanese Martial Arts, we hear of ninjas who run one hundred miles per day, becoming invincible, performing incredible feats.

Orasyon, Bulong and Dasal are Filipino spiritual practices deeply based in Christianity, combined with Tantric tradition. Many of us may be confused by all these paths, however, in reality, this only broadens our understanding of the universality of each and every religious or spiritual discipline. This is the true essence of universal enlightenment and universal understanding. As my master has said of religions; They are all flowers in one beautiful garden.

"ORASYON is a state of consciousness. It works like magic when your mind and body is pure".

XX.

ORASYON/DASAL

O Mahal Kung, Bathala
Bigyan mo po ako ng lakas para itupad and Misyon dito
Sa Mundo
Ipakita mo po ang ilaw sa daan ng kataasan
Ituro mo po ako sa daan para Maliwanagan
Bigyan daan ang aking lakas para sa inyong Banal na
Dharma
Huwag akong maligaw sa aking landas
Huwag pong sariling egom at aking isip
Mag-hadlang sa tunay na disciplo ninyo
Huwag po akong mabigo sa pagkatunay
Na Missionario ninyo dito sa mundo

Mahal kung Bathala
Ikaw lang ang makapayarihan
Magbigay galang ako sa inyo
Pahalikin po ninyo ako sa inyong paa

Akoy inyong Utusan
Pabayaan ninyo po akung magsilbi sa inyong banal na
Kautusan
Pabayaan ninyo pong ang aking pag–iisip
Magbigay linaw sa inyong banal na kalagayan
Akoy walang kailangan kundi ang inyong
Banal na pag mamahal at Dharma

Mahal kung Diyos
Kunin ninyo akung utusan
Pabayaan ninyo akong maglingkod ng aking
Isip at puso
Ikaw ang aking lakas
Ikaw na nagbigay diwa sa lahat
Iko'y mapa sa inyo
Kunin ninyo Ako
Aum Santo
Aum Santo
Aum

ORASYON/DASAL

(ENGLISH TRANSLATION)

Oh Divine Guru,
Give me enough strength to fulfill your mission on this earth.
Show me the path to Enlightenment.
Give me enough guidance to understand the way.
Direct my will and power to the Divine Purpose.
Let me not become distracted from my destiny.
Let not my ego and my will ham per my growth as your true follower.
Let me not fail you as your missionary in this world.
Protect me from worldly temptations.

Oh Divine Guru,
You alone can make things happen.
I bow to you.
I kiss your Lotus feet.

As your servant, let me serve your divine command.
Let my mind and my thoughts envision your Divine
Presence.
Let me deserve nothing else but your Divine Love and
Purpose.

Oh Divine Guru,
Take me as your humble servant.
Let me serve you with my heart and mind.
You, as the source of my strength,
You, as the source of my existence,
Let me be with you.
Aum Shanti,
Aum Shanti,
Peace, peace, peace.

Originated in Bagiu City, Philippines, revised May 1972
in Vanarasi, India and finalized December 1983, Assisi,
Rome, Italy.

XXI.

ENLIGHTENMENT

It is my persona l realization that each and everyone of us is born for a purpose. Finding this purpose, in whatever form or path, is termed seeking. Finding our individual path and practicing it is what we call discipline. Seeking, and, finally, practicing our personal and social belief, is our way of life.

Maintaining our way and realizing our purpose is what we call Enlightenment. Let us not become distracted from the true path of Enlightenment nor discouraged as we walk it, for we are all heading toward the same goal. We only differ in the manner and level of in sight. There is good and bad in all things. There are evils and virtues everywhere. We should not seek to be good or to be bad, but seek our purpose, maximizing our potential and continuously growing until we find our destiny.

Destiny and Enlightenment have something in common. They are both a stage of fulfillment, however, destiny can change for better or for worse. Enlightenment, on the other hand, is a stage of spiritual realization and it remains forever positive. Enlightenment is the stage at which everything becomes simpler and practical. It is as if nature works alongside you. Everything happens naturally and successfully. That is why an Enlightened being can be at war, and, at the same time, be at peace. He or she can be poor but find contentment and happiness. He or she can be wealthy, yet also find balance and simplicity. This means that every human being can be enlightened. Whatever we do, we can attain enlightenment.

There are four stages of enlightenment.

1) Confusion – we are lo st and confused,

2) Seeking – we seek to find ways – paths, teacher or knowledge of discipline,

3) Finding – at this stage, the seeker finds his or her path and Master, but retains ego, "a feeling of, 'I am the best'"

4) Enlightenment – when the discipline becomes a living philosophy. He or she becomes an example of the way. There is no longer an ego.

XXII

CONCLUSION

To Meditate:

(1) Preparation

— Eyes closed, relax, sit with spine straight, feel your breathing.

(2) Withdrawal

— Imagine yourself alone, feel your entire body. Imagine a light around your body. Light entering your toes, shins, knee, thigh, spine, stomach, arms, shoulder, face, head and finally, the center of your forehead.

(3) Concentration (Focusing)

— Visualize a light in your forehead, Breathe in and breathe out... relax. Repeat your mantra — orasyon — in the inhalation and exhalation.

(4) Meditation

– Bring the light deeply within you. Merge yourself (ego) with the light and feel the meaning of your Orasyon. "I am with the universal energy... oneness".

(5) Clarity

– This is the stage of Enlightenment or Self-realization. It is the stage of the Spiritual Warrior.

ABOUT THE AUTHOR

Shishir Inocalla began his Martial Arts training in early childhood. Since that time, he has balanced his Mastery of the Martial Arts with an extensive spiritual training.

He was taught by his parents Filipino Orasyones. Before he was fifteen years of age, he travelled to India, to study meditation under a leading master. He entered a monastery, followed by service in an orphanage, before leaving for the eastern continent.

He was awarded the title Acharya, meaning teacher-by-example, and Datu, a Spiritual Warrior.

He has travelled worldwide, giving demonstrations and seminars in Filipino Martial Arts, Arnis, and in Meditation. Now living in Vancouver, Canada, Datu Inocalla administers an Arnis Martial Arts Center and continues his study and writing.

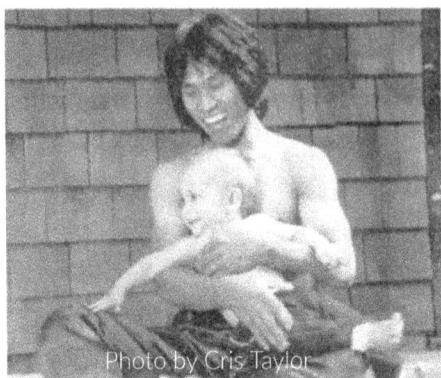

Photo by Cris Taylor

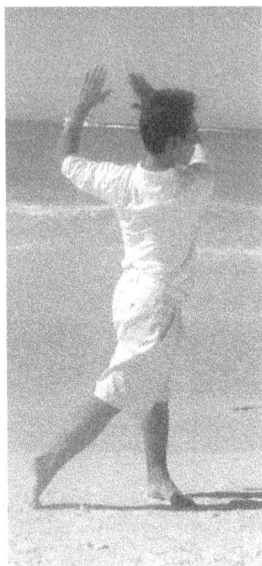

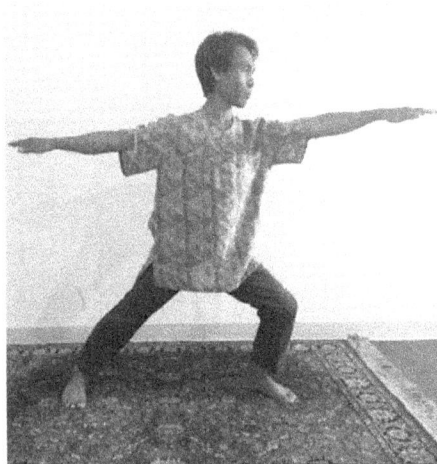

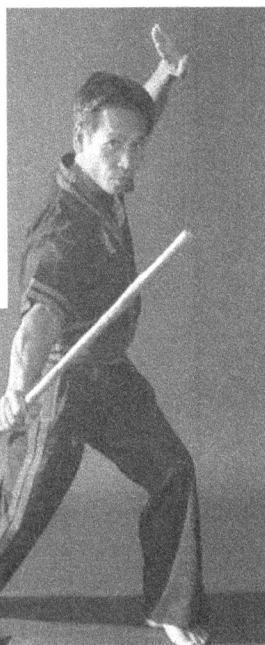

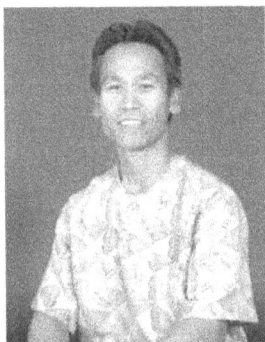

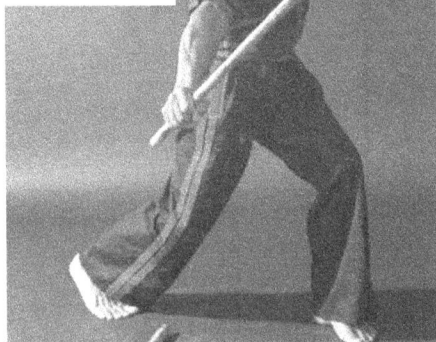

www.ingramcontent.com/pod-product-compliance
Lightning Source LLC
Chambersburg PA
CBHW022337280326
41934CB00006B/670